The Tuskegee
Veterans Hospital
and Its Black Physicians

The Tuskegee Veterans Hospital and Its Black Physicians
The Early Years

MARY KAPLAN

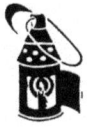

McFarland & Company, Inc., Publishers
Jefferson, North Carolina

LIBRARY OF CONGRESS CATALOGUING-IN-PUBLICATION DATA

Names: Kaplan, Mary, author.
Title: The Tuskegee Veterans Hospital and its Black physicians : the early years / Mary Kaplan.
Description: Jefferson, North Carolina : McFarland & Company, Inc., 2016 | Includes bibliographical references and index.
Identifiers: LCCN 2016017901 | ISBN 9781476662985 (softcover : acid free paper) ∞
Subjects: LCSH: Tuskegee Veterans Hospital. | African American veterans—Medical care—History—20th century. | African American physicians—History—20th century. | Military hospitals—United States—History—20th century.
Classification: LCC UH474.5.T87 K37 2016 | DDC 362.11086/970976149—dc23
LC record available at https://lccn.loc.gov/2016017901

BRITISH LIBRARY CATALOGUING DATA ARE AVAILABLE

ISBN (print) 978-1-4766-6298-5
ISBN (ebook) 978-1-4766-2548-5

© 2016 Mary Kaplan. All rights reserved

No part of this book may be reproduced or transmitted in any form or by any means, electronic or mechanical, including photocopying or recording, or by any information storage and retrieval system, without permission in writing from the publisher.

Front cover: the Tuskegee Veterans Hospital, Tuskegee, Alabama, in a photograph by Mary Kaplan, 2008

Printed in the United States of America

McFarland & Company, Inc., Publishers
 Box 611, Jefferson, North Carolina 28640
  www.mcfarlandpub.com

Acknowledgments

I am grateful to those who helped me in my quest to document the "other legacy" of Tuskegee and the important role that its veterans hospital and medical staff played in the medical care of black veterans. I was fortunate to be able to talk to family members of some of the physicians featured in this book, who gave meaning to the archival materials and historical accounts. Shortly after I began my research, I discovered that a relative of Toussaint Tildon was a student in one of my classes. Nancy Braye-Washington made arrangements for me to meet her father, James T. Braye, who was a great-nephew of Dr. Tildon. Arriving in Tuskegee, I was instructed to drive to a convenience store and look for an old green Cadillac. I spent the rest of the day driving through rural Tuskegee in that Cadillac with Mr. Braye as my guide. Having worked at the Tuskegee VA as the director of human relations during the infamous syphilis study, he was able to provide firsthand knowledge about the hospital's involvement as well as information about its medical staff. He also gave me a tour of the hospital and helped me gain access to its library. Other family members who gave generously of their time and provided me with valuable insight into their families and their experiences in Tuskegee were Dr. George Branche, III, June G. Branche, Frances King, and Dr. Judith King-Calnek. A special thank you also goes to Ted Gup, journalist, and to John L. Fuller, grandson of Dr. Solomon Carter Fuller.

Thanks are also due to the staffs of the libraries and archives that were particularly helpful. A special thank you goes to A'Llyn Ettien at the Boston University Alumni Medical Library Archives, Dana Chandler and Cheryl Ferguson and their staff at the Tuskegee Archives, Tuskegee University, Alana Love, director of the library at the Tuskegee

Acknowledgments

Veterans Hospital, and the staff at the Francis A. Countway Library of Medicine, Harvard Medical Library, the History of Medicine Archives, the National Library of Medicine, and the Library of Congress Manuscript Division. They were a great resource and source of enthusiasm and support for my research as well as a constant reminder that, in this era of online technology, the value of working with a dedicated staff person cannot be overstated.

My sincere appreciation to Shelby Forbes for her work in formatting the manuscript and to the Pasco Camera Exchange for enhancing the images of the people in this work.

My family is a constant source of support and encouragement and it is exciting to see my four granddaughters grow into bookworms. My husband, Roy, has been my partner in life and constant supporter for half a century. I'm grateful for his love, encouragement and unwavering belief in my work.

Table of Contents

Acknowledgments — v
Preface — 1
Introduction — 4

1. Threats, Fear and Triumph: The Opening of the Tuskegee Veterans Hospital — 23
2. Health Care for Black Veterans — 50
3. Responding to the Call for Black Physicians at the Tuskegee Hospital — 64
4. Fuller's Trainees — 76
5. The Practice of Medicine by Black Physicians in the Jim Crow South — 81
6. The Tuskegee Veterans Hospital: Challenges, Successes and Scandal — 89
7. 1986: Thirty-Seven Years Later — 122

Chapter Notes — 129
Bibliography — 139
Index — 147

Preface

More than eighty years have passed since the first American hospital built to treat the country's black veterans opened its doors. During this time, the country experienced many challenges and advances in the march toward freedom and equal rights for African Americans. From the great migration during the World War I period and the race riots that followed the end of the war; the achievements of black writers and artists during the Harlem Renaissance of the 1920s; the Civil Rights era resulting in the Freedom Rides of 1947 and *Brown v. Board of Education* in 1954; the urban riots of the 1960s; and the passage of the 1964 Civil Rights Act to the election of America's first black president in 2008, there has been progress in the reach for racial equality, although bigotry and discrimination continue to exist in American society.

In many ways, the history of the Tuskegee Veterans Hospital reflects the struggle for racial equality in the United States. To enable the reader to understand the military segregation that was a symbol of the rampant discrimination encountered, this book provides a history of the treatment of blacks in the military from the Revolutionary War through World War II. The inability of black veterans to receive the same access to and quality of treatment as white veterans was just another example of the institutional racism that existed in the military, reinforced by the country's laws and belief in the supremacy of the Anglo-Saxon race. African Americans were refused admission to most hospitals, and when they were admitted, received inferior care in segregated wards.

This book is an account of the United States Veterans Administration's efforts to construct and develop a medical facility designed to

Preface

provide treatment to black veterans. When the Tuskegee hospital opened in 1923, there were many in the Veterans Bureau who believed that black medical professionals were not competent to staff the facility and it was decided that, with the exception of nurse aides, orderlies, attendants, and laborers, the hospital personnel would be white. This book describes the struggle to integrate the hospital staff. The effort to recruit and train black professional staff who were approved by the Civil Service Commission was a formidable one given the difficulties encountered by many African Americans in obtaining education and advanced training in medicine, and gaining acceptance in the medical field. Today, black physicians can be found on the faculties of major American medical colleges, on the staff of most hospitals and clinics, in influential positions at the state and federal levels, and making important contributions in medical and scientific research.

I first learned about the black physicians who joined the Tuskegee Veterans Hospital staff and broke the color barrier while doing research for my biography of Dr. Solomon Carter Fuller, *Solomon Carter Fuller: Where My Caravan Has Rested*, which explores the life of the man who is considered American's first black psychiatrist. My intent in writing about Dr. Fuller's life and accomplishments was to make known his contributions to research in Alzheimer's disease and mental illness as well as to the practice of psychiatry. In my ten years of research, which included archival research and interviews with his family and friends, I found that, in addition to his medical and scientific achievements, Dr. Fuller was a man with strong family and professional values and who, despite the obstacles of racism, wanted to serve his country. His efforts to enlist in World War I as a neuropsychiatrist to the military were rejected; his race would be an obstacle in attaining military rank. When approached three years later by the Veterans Administration and asked to direct the mental health treatment program at the new Tuskegee Veterans Hospital, Dr. Fuller declined the offer, but did agree to train a small group of black medical school graduates in neuropsychiatry.

George Branche, Harvey Davis, Simon O. Johnson, and Toussaint Tildon, graduates of prominent Boston medical schools, received training under the supervision of Dr. Fuller before accepting staff positions at Tuskegee. In addition to describing the events that led to the opening

Preface

of the Tuskegee Veterans Hospital, the book follows the careers and contributions of this small group of well trained and dedicated physicians who played significant roles in the hospital's development as a treatment center for black veterans. The hospital's important contributions to research and medicine are documented as well as its involvement in what was to be one of the largest scandals in medical research—the Tuskegee Syphilis Study.

The material for this book has been collected from archival collections as well as from interviews with family members and Tuskegee Veterans Hospital employees. Their experiences and recollections provide unique insights into a community of black professionals living and working in the Deep South under the pressures of Jim Crow segregation who demonstrated remarkable resilience and found ways to achieve success in the field of medicine.

Introduction

African Americans served in every American war and when given the opportunity, to fight performed well on many battlefields. In order to understand and appreciate the significance of the Tuskegee Veterans Hospital and the role that it played in providing quality and accessible medical care to black veterans, it is essential to have a sense of the history of the treatment of African Americans in the United States military.

The absence of black people's names on war documents makes it difficult to estimate the number of African Americans who served their country in early wars. They were deliberately left off of military rolls, and only a few were mentioned. When listed, they were often identified only by their common slave names or as a "Negro, name unknown" or "mulatto waiting boy." Frederick Douglass wrote:

> He was already in the army as a waiter, and in that capacity there was no objection to him, and so it was thought that as this was the case, the feeling which tolerated him as a waiter would not seriously object if he should be admitted to the army as a laborer. This was the first step in employing Negroes in the United States service. The second step was to give them a peculiar costume which should distinguish them from soldiers, and yet mark them as a part of the loyal force. As the eyes of the loyal administration still further opened, it was proposed to give these laborers something better than spades and shovels with which to defend themselves in cases of emergency. Still later it was proposed to make them soldiers, but soldiers without the blue uniform, soldiers with a mark upon them to show that they were inferior to other soldiers—soldiers with a badge of degradation upon them. However, once in the army as a laborer, once there with a red shirt on his back and a pistol in his belt, the Negro was not long in appearing on the field as a soldier. But still, he was not to be a soldier in the sense, and on equal footing, with white soldiers.[1]

Introduction

By joining the military, African Americans felt that they could escape the repression and discrimination that they faced in American society. There was an element of respect and self-esteem associated with being a member of the armed forces. But, as history would demonstrate, helping to defend their country did not gain them acceptance within the military nor did it bring them full citizenship when they returned home. Only as wars became broader in scope and longer in duration, requiring the support and participation of America's entire population, did Jim Crow laws relax their hold on the armed forces and other elements of society.[2]

White colonial militiamen used blacks for manual labor, only trusting them with weapons and ammunition when threatened with an Indian attack or invasion. Prior to the beginning of the Revolutionary War, African Americans had served as Minutemen, volunteers who defended local towns. The colonies made no reference to race as a criterion for membership, but by 1639 Virginia had enacted legislation excluding "Negroes" from being provided with arms or ammunition. New England colonies, following Virginia's lead, soon began to ban African Americans from militia organizations. Despite the restrictions placed on blacks in the militia during the colonial period, free blacks were usually permitted to enlist in New England and the central colonies but denied leadership roles.

During the French and Indian War, which began in 1753 over the boundaries of French and English settlements, blacks served as scouts, wagoners, and laborers for the English. In addition, black militiamen served with independent colonial units from Pennsylvania, South Carolina, Virginia, New York, New Jersey, and Massachusetts. Throughout the year, until the war's end in 1754, African Americans distinguished themselves in battles at Fort Duquesne, Fort Cumberland, and the Plains of Abraham outside Quebec.

When the American Revolution began, as many as 5000 blacks joined local and state militias.[3] Slaves had nothing to lose by enlisting and they saw it as a way to escape the degradation and suffering of plantation life. They fought at Lexington, Concord, and Bunker Hill, where many were recognized as heroes. Pressured by patriot leaders, who feared that the enlistment of African American soldiers would encourage slaves to leave their masters, and Southern white politicians,

Introduction

who warned against allowing blacks to be armed with guns, George Washington was forced to forbid all blacks from fighting when he organized the Continental army on July 9, 1775. The ban not only included the enlistment of new black soldiers but also forbade the reenlistment of black men who had served in earlier battles. It wasn't long before similar restrictions were enacted by all thirteen states. These restrictions were lifted when the governor of Virginia, the Earl of Dunmore, influenced by a growing shortage of fighting men and seeing the potential for new recruits, issued a proclamation on November 7, 1775, which stated: "And I do hereby further declare all indentured servant Negroes of others, free, that are able and willing to bear arms, they joining His Majesty's Troops, as soon as may be, for the more speedily reducing the Colony to a proper sense of their duty, to His Majesty's crown and dignity."[4] Within one month of the recruitment proclamation, almost 300 African Americans had joined the British army's "Ethiopian Regiment," wearing uniforms inscribed with "Liberty to Slaves."

As the war dragged on and the continental army was reduced to 6,000 volunteers, Washington eliminated the ban and allowed freed blacks who had fought in the early campaigns to reenlist. The Southern states of Delaware, Maryland, Virginia, and North Carolina reluctantly followed suit and began enlisting black men. Although slave participation was prohibited, slaves did participate—many substituting for their masters who did not want to serve. When the war ended, approximately 5,000 African Americans had served in the colonial army, participating in most major battles and winning honors and praise from their commanders. While some who were slaves were freed and some received land grants for service, the majority of blacks who had served in the military were returned to slavery.

Restrictions on blacks in the military continued under the Militia Act, passed in 1792, which limited service in all state militias except in North Carolina to "each and every free and able-bodied white male citizen of the respective states."[5] In 1798, Negroes, mulattos and Indians were prohibited from joining the Marines by Secretary of War Henry Knox, and Negroes and mulattoes were barred from the navy by Secretary of the Navy Benjamin Stoddard. The ban on black enlistment in the navy was disregarded during the War of 1812, which proved, for

Introduction

the most part, to be a naval war with fleets engaged at sea and on the Great Lakes. Black sailors, with their Revolutionary War experience and their ability to obtain shipping jobs, were a valuable source of manpower and constituted from 10 to 20 percent of most ships' crews.

The black soldier continued to be excluded in land battles, with their attempts to volunteer refused in most states. Several months after the War of 1812 erupted, an invasion by British troops near New Orleans prompted militia general Andrew Jackson to assemble troops near Crescent City to go to battle. His army was a mix of Southern frontiersmen and dandies, pirates, Creoles, and slaves, and included two battalions of 600 free blacks, commanded by several black officers. When the British invaded the Chesapeake in the spring of 1813, the British offered the promise of freedom in Canada or the British West Indies to slaves in return for their help in battle. In response, a number of African Americans joined the British army and participated in the burning of Washington, D.C., and the attack on Baltimore the following year. Threatened by possible attacks by the British army on nearby Philadelphia and New York, the New York state legislature authorized black regiments, offering freedom to slaves who enlisted and compensation to slave owners. In 1814, approximately 2000 blacks, slave and free were enlisted in two of the state's regiments.

On January 8, 1815, under Jackson, for the first time in history, American troops were led by African Americans at the Battle of New Orleans on January 8, 1815. Jackson had the highest praise for his black soldiers and he promised freedom to his slave recruits as well as promises to the freed blacks of pay, bounties, and land grants equal to those of his white soldiers. Following the battle, General Jackson reneged on the promise of bounties and land for his black soldiers as well as his promise of freedom for the slaves, insisting that he did not have the power to free "another man's property." In a speech to white compatriots in a New Orleans tavern, he announced: "Before a slave of mine should go free I would put him in a barn and burn him alive. Never arm another set of colored people. We have fooled them now, but will they will be fooled again with this example before them."[6] This declaration infuriated one African American soldier and veteran of the Revolutionary War, James Roberts, who took out his pistol and attempted to shoot Jackson. But, what Roberts did not know was that the day

Introduction

after the battle, Jackson had confiscated the weapons of all his black soldiers and ordered their ammunition removed.

When New Orleans held its parades honoring the key battle victory, no black units, including the two heroic battalions of freed blacks, were allowed to march.

By 1820, the army had returned to its "whites only" policy and the navy had limited black recruitment to less than 5 percent. When the Civil War began in 1861, African Americans who wanted to enlist were rejected. Recognizing that the future of slavery would be influenced by the outcome of the war between the North and the South, black men volunteered their services and in some states formed their own military companies and began to drill. Following the attack on Fort Sumter, a black employee of the U.S. Senate wrote a letter to Secretary of War Simon Cameron, volunteering the services of black men in Washington. "I desire to inform you that I know of some 300 reliable colored free citizens of this city who desire to enter the service for the defense of the city." Cameron replied: "This department has no intention at the present to call into service of the government any colored soldiers."[7]

The First Confiscation Act was passed on August 6, 1861, freeing captured slaves used by the Confederate army. A year later, following the Battle of Antietam, the Emancipation Proclamation was issued, marking the beginning of the end of slavery. This document, along with the Second Confiscation Act and the Militia Act passed by Congress in 1862, allowed President Lincoln to enlist black recruits to suppress the Southern rebellion. Motivated by the call to not only fight for their freedom, but to also prove that they deserved it, nearly 40,000 blacks enlisted. Although black troops were allowed to serve, regiments remained segregated. The War Department created the Bureau of Colored Troops and the Union army refused to integrate black men into all-white regiments. Most black troops were commanded by white officers, many who regarded the men as "niggers" who were unfit for combat. The first black unit consisted of 500 men, most of them runaway slaves from Missouri and Arkansas.[8] They entered combat in October 1862 against a Confederate army in Missouri, holding off an attack until reinforcements arrived. Soon after the successful battle, the black unit became the 1st Kansas Colored Infantry.

Introduction

It took an extra measure of courage for blacks to fight in this war because of the Confederacy's threat that black soldiers who were captured would be treated as insurrectionists, meaning they could be subjected to torture and brutalities under the pretense of patriotic duty. Confederate commanders and soldiers were enraged at having to fight black troops and refused to recognize them as legitimate soldiers. After the war, a Congressional panel heard testimony from twenty-one witnesses who reported that at the battle at Fort Pillow, Tennessee, on April 12, 1864, a rebel force stormed a Union garrison on the Mississippi defended by 570 soldiers, nearly half of them black, yelling, "Kill all the niggers!" It was established that at least 300 Union troops, mostly black, were massacred after they surrendered. When news of the Fort Pillow massacre spread, it fueled the emotion and determination of black troops, who charged into battle yelling, "Remember Fort Pillow!"[9]

Despite the fact the black soldiers were paid only $10 per month, compared to the $13 paid to their white counterparts and had an extra $3 per month deducted from their pay for clothing while whites received an extra $3.50 per month for clothing, they continued to distinguish themselves in battle, performing many acts of heroism that led to twelve Medals of Honor. In protest against this inequality and indignity, troops of the 54th Massachusetts regiment went without pay for a year, and in January 1864, equal pay was finally won.

The success of the colored troops in the Civil War led President Andrew Johnson to recommend on July 28, 1866, that they be incorporated into the regular army. Through an act of Congress, legislation was passed to create six all African American army units. These units served until the end of the century at forts along the country's western frontier, where they continued to encounter racial disparities, such as the inability to rise to the rank of officer, inferior (usually castoffs) equipment and horses, and poor living quarters.

Black sailors, who had been in the U.S. navy since its creation in the 1790s and who served in integrated crews, also encountered widespread discrimination and exploitation during the Civil War. Often treated with contempt by white officers, they were referred to as "black dog," "black bitches," and "God-damned nigger." The estimated 30,000

Introduction

black sailors who served in the Union navy were paid less than white sailors and, with the exception of a few who achieved positions of engineers and pilots, were usually assigned to the boiler room or as stewards to white officers.

As the military situation deteriorated in the South, the Confederate congress voted to enlist 300,000 black men in March 1865, despite the opposition of many white Southerners. This move to enroll and emancipate black troops was influenced by General Robert E. Lee: "My own opinion is that we should employ them without delay. They possess the physical qualities in an eminent degree. Long habits of obedience and subordination, coupled with moral influence which in our country the white man possesses over the black, furnish an excellent foundation for that discipline which is the best guarantee of military efficiency."[10]

There were several reasons that most Southern leaders did not accept the concept of blacks serving in the Confederate army or navy. First, they thought that the Southern Negroes were loyal to the North and its stand on emancipation. The fear of the wrath of armed blacks was a concern to many white citizens in the South. Second, the South's economic base was dependent on slavery and if the slaves became soldiers, this would have a direct effect on the economy. A further consideration was the strong aversion of white Southerners to fight side by side on an equal standing with Negroes.[11]

In an effort to secure just and fair treatment for black soldiers, Frederick Douglass, a former slave who became a symbol for freedom for African Americans, met with President Lincoln.

> Several months before I had been very successful in getting men to enlist, but that now it was not easy to induce the colored men to enter the service, because there was feeling among them that the government did not, in several respects, deal fairly with them. Mr. Lincoln asked me to state particulars which I wished to bring to his attention. First, that colored soldiers ought to receive the same wages as those paid to white soldiers. Second, that colored soldiers ought to receive the same protection when taken prisoners, and be exchanged as readily and on the same terms as any other prisoners, and if Jefferson Davis should shoot or hang colored soldiers in cold blood the United States government should, without delay, retaliate in kind and degree upon Confederate prisoners in its hands. Third, when colored soldiers, seeking "the bubble reputation at the cannon's mouth," performed great and uncommon service on the

Introduction

battlefield, they should be rewarded by distinction and promotion precisely as white soldiers are rewarded for like services."[12]

Douglass' sons, Lewis and Charles, responded to their father's call to enlist and joined the 54th Massachusetts Volunteer Infantry. While Douglass did not achieve the promise of equality for black soldiers that he had hoped for, he was heartened by Lincoln's concern and expressed new hope when the Emancipation Proclamation was issued on January 1, 1863: "For my own part, I took the proclamation, first and last, for a little more than it purported, saw in its spirit a life and power far beyond its letter. Its meaning to me was the entire abolition of slavery, wherever the evil could be reached by the federal arm, and I saw that its moral power would extend much further."[13]

Upon closer and more critical examination, the proclamation was found to be limited in its promise of liberty for all of the country's citizens. It only abolished slavery where it did not already exist and its directive was confined within specific geographical and military boundaries. Only those slaves in Confederate breakaway states were freed in an attempt to cripple the South's economy and to induce slaves to rebel and enlist in the Union army.[14] The document was inspired by military necessity and would become inoperative when the conflict was over.

Although many of the 180,000 black soldiers who fought for the Union were relegated to support services, the army gave black soldiers the right to attain officer rank in considerable number for the first time and abolitionist Union officers established schools for black troops. This was a significant achievement at a time when black civilians were not afforded the ability to work in the same occupations as whites or receive equal pay.

Forty thousand black soldiers died in the Civil War.[15] For many, their deaths were due to poor equipment, bad medical care, and the "no quarter" policy followed by the Confederate forces. An exception to the battlefield tradition of accepting the surrender of enemy soldiers and extending protection to the wounded was issued by Confederate president Jefferson Davis, who ordered all black soldiers caught in uniform to be considered escaped slaves and returned to their masters. Davis also declared that white officers leading black soldiers would be executed if captured. In practice, the usual fate for black soldiers was often a merciless death in battle or, if captured, execution afterward.[16]

Introduction

African Americans served in all military branches from 1864 until the end of the Civil War. Despite the fact that over 129 black infantry regiments were raised in addition to seven cavalry regiments, twelve heavy artillery regiments, five engineer regiments, and ten batteries of light artillery, only one company of thirty-five black men was organized by the end of the war. After the Civil War, when the army reduced its troops to less than 30,000, there was an attempt by Congressional Democrats to eliminate black soldiers from their ranks. The Army Reorganization Act of 1869 succeeded in keeping military enlistment open to black men and established four all-black regiments. Those regiments, the 9th and 10th Cavalry and the 24th and 25th Infantry, with close to 12,500 black soldiers, served for the next three decades on the western frontier. The decision to move the black troops to western posts was influenced by the tensions between the white Southerners and the black soldiers, who refused to revert to prewar servility.[17] Most of the black regiments were assigned to west Texas and to the New Mexico and Arizona territories because of the belief that they could tolerate heat better than the white soldiers due to their African ancestry. One out of every five of the soldiers in these territories was black, but it was not until 1877 that a Negro officer, Henry O. Flipper, the first black graduate from West Point, was assigned to the 10th Cavalry.[18] Some black troops were sent to Colorado, Kansas, and the Dakotas, where they were forced to endure subzero temperatures and blizzards without adequate housing or supplies. While the army provided its white soldiers with dried fruit, canned and fresh vegetables, black troops were fed spoiled beef, moldy bread and canned peas. Black regiments were supplied with old horses, allotted used weapons and equipment and were often forced to sleep in outdoors in tents, while the white soldiers lived in barracks. A black soldier could expect little mercy, even for minor offenses, at the hands of a court-martial. A dishonorable discharge and one year sentence of hard labor was the customary penalty for drunkenness while on duty.

In their encounters with the Plains Indians, the black soldiers' performance impressed their adversaries, who gave them the name "Buffalo Soldiers." The Indians associated the hair of black men with the rugged coat of the buffalo, which they considered to be a sacred animal. The 10th Cavalry, considering it a symbol of respect, adopted

Introduction

the buffalo as their unit emblem. Although the four black regiments repeatedly fought unfriendly Indians from the late 1860s to the early 1890s, there were several instances where the 9th and 10th Cavalry protected members of the Kiowa, Chickasaw, Cherokee, and Sioux tribes from attacks by Texas Rangers and other hostile groups.

Black veterans of the Civil War continued their commitment to serving their country by forming militias and paramilitary organizations after the war. Faced with limited access to military training, a group of officers from black regiments established separate training schools for African American soldiers.[19] In addition to providing martial instruction, the training schools held annual weeklong encampments that enabled the black state militiamen to interact with the citizens they pledged to protect. The two companies that comprised the 1st Alabama Battalion, Mobile's Gilmer Rifles and Montgomery's Capital City Guards, gained national recognition and were later invited to join the white battalions at the Alabama State Troop training camps in Mobile. Despite the success of integrated encampments, mock battles, and parades in Alabama and in other Southern states such as Virginia and Georgia, there was increasing concern on the part of many white leaders and public officials that these well respected black soldiers presented a danger to the self-ascribed white identity of Southern men as being the only ones capable of "civility and restraint." The rise of the Southern Redemption movement, intent on obstructing the political equality and social advancement of African Americans, resulted in the disbanding of black state militia units by 1905.

Although the climate of hate and racial prejudice intensified in the years following the Civil War, blacks were still willing to fight for their country during the Spanish-American War. In both the North and the South, blacks experienced segregation of public facilities and the South used Black Codes, literacy tests, and poll taxes to disenfranchise blacks. The 1896 *Plessy v. Ferguson* ruling by the Supreme Court established the "separate but equal" concept that made it legal for a double standard in society that allowed separate accommodations for blacks and whites in the military.[20]

Amid this political climate, the military, along with many white Americans, felt that it was morally and militarily unacceptable to place

Introduction

black officers in command of any black regiments. The only remaining black state militia unit in the South, the 1st Alabama, well respected for its reputation for flawless drill and discipline, was among those state volunteer units that were called up by the United States government in the war with Spain. When Major Mims and Captain C. J. Harlbert were asked to step down to enable their posts to be filled with white officers from the U.S. army, most of the unit remained loyal to their black officers and refused to disband or join another company, despite orders from the Alabama governor, Joseph F. Johnston. A new unit, the 3rd Alabama Volunteers, was eventually formed, made up of African Americans from throughout the state and led by a white officer. Those black soldiers who remained with the 1st Alabama were not permitted to fight in Cuba and were mustered out in 1905.[21]

Twenty-two black sailors were among the 266 troops killed in the explosion of the *Maine* in Havana Harbor on February 15, 1898.[22] Following the attack, sixteen volunteer black regiments were mobilized to fight overseas. This marked the first time that African Americans were sent to foreign posts to defend the United States. Many black regiments, including the Buffalo Soldiers, fought with Teddy Roosevelt's troops to secure victories at San Juan Hill and other battlegrounds. Black troops assembled alongside white troops in Georgia and Florida before departing for Cuba. For the first time in American military history, black men were permitted to command black volunteer units, but all the higher ranking officers continued to be white men. In Cuba, soldiers of the black 10th Cavalry fought next to Cuban rebels, many of whom were also black. Although many of the black volunteer units never saw combat, the four regiments of regular black troops performed well, with four black American privates earning the Medal of Honor. At the end of the hostilities, members of the black 24th Infantry stayed in Cuba to work in yellow fever hospitals and about half of them contracted the disease.

There was the initial fanfare of parades and speeches when the black soldiers arrived back in the United States, but they soon found themselves again facing the daily challenges of a racist society. When sent to the Philippines in 1899 as part of a United States effort to suppress the insurrection of Emilio Aguinaldo, many members of the black regiments started to identify with the Filipinos who were oppressed by

Introduction

the imperialistic Spanish.[23] They saw the movement as another fight for freedom by people of color and a large number of black soldiers defected, with many joining the enemy insurgents. Those who were caught and tried were eventually hung or committed to serving life sentences with hard labor.

Racial bias continued to escalate at home and in the army, where segregation had become the accepted rule. Black soldiers also encountered prejudice when stationed in the South. The situation exploded when three companies of the 24th Infantry were sent to Fort Brown, located near Brownsville, Texas. Conflict between the black soldiers and the town began when a local custom official pistol-whipped a black soldier for not moving off the sidewalk when a white woman approached. Several other incidents, including a charge of attempted abduction of a white woman by a black soldier and an allegation that "the nigger soldiers" were responsible for a shooting spree despite the lack of evidence, led to an order by President Roosevelt to move the black battalion to Oklahoma. At the same time, Roosevelt demanded that the perpetrators come forward or he would have all three companies dishonorably discharged and prohibited from reenlisting. When no one confessed, it was determined to be a conspiracy of silence and all 167 soldiers were dismissed without a hearing.[24]

When a special board of inquiry met in 1908 to review the dismissals, no decision was reached. A year later, Ohio senator Joseph Foraker arranged for an army rehearing, with five generals taking testimony. Eighty-two soldiers testified and seventy others who applied to be heard were refused. Based on the accepted testimonies pointing to guilt, on April 6, 1910, the generals decided that everyone was guilty and all but fourteen soldiers would not be permitted to reenlist. It took sixty-two years for the injustice to be overturned, when Augustus Hawkins, an African American congressman from California, initiated a Defense Department review of the case. On April 28, 1972, the secretary of the army, acknowledging that "egregious errors" had been made, issued honorable discharges to all 167 soldiers. Only one, Dorsie Willis, eighty-six years old, was still alive. He was awarded $25,000 from Congress and given the right to receive treatment at veterans facilities. After his dismissal from the army, Willis had spent the remainder of his life sweeping floors and shining shoes. When notified

Introduction

of the reversal of his military discharge, he remarked, "That dishonorable discharge kept me from improving my station. Only God knows what it did to others."[25]

The event of World War I saw the need for extensive manpower, forcing the military to reconsider the recruitment of black soldiers. By 1917, institutionalized racism had limited opportunities for African Americans and segregation was the norm in society and in the military. Although denied their full freedom for which the United States fought, large numbers of African Americans volunteered to fight for their country, hoping that their military contribution would demonstrate their desire and ability to participate fully in society. Worried about the increasing number of blacks in the military, policy makers had limited the number of African Americans in the military to 10 percent, reflecting the percentage in the nation's population. While most branches of the military were integrated, the Marine corps continued to exclude blacks. Those Marines, who found themselves working alongside black members of army stevedore battalions in France, complained of having to work with "niggers."[26]

As in previous wars, provisions for African American troops were inadequate and inferior. Black stevedores who traveled by ship to France were forced to sleep below deck with little or no ventilation. Some soldiers were given old Civil War uniforms to wear and lacked coats and shoes. Up to thirty men were often housed in 16-by-16-foot tents with no access to bathing facilities, while white servicemen slept in barracks. Their food was served outdoors, frequently freezing in the winter before they could eat it. During the winter of 1917–1918, over twenty black soldiers at Camp Alexandria, Virginia, froze to death in their tents.[27]

Approximately 380,000 African Americans were conscripted for service, including more than 1,200 officers commissioned to lead in combat. Over 200,000 black soldiers served in France, most in support units. Two African American divisions (92nd and 93rd), comprised of 40,000 troops, were formed and joined the Allied Expeditionary Force (AEF) in France. The AEF had campaigned to keep blacks out of the war and most of its officers were Southern whites who did their best to demoralize the black soldiers. The 92nd Division saw little action and were used mainly in the war's last assault on the Hindenburg line.

Introduction

When the 93rd was transferred to the French command, the AEF issued a guide to understanding American blacks.

> Although a citizen of the United States, the black man is regarded by white Americans as an inferior being. The black is constantly being censured for his tendency toward undue familiarity. The vices of the Negro are a constant menace to the American who has to repress them strongly. We must prevent the rise of any pronounced degree of intimacy between French officers and black officers. We must not eat with them or seek to talk with them outside of the arrangements of military service.[28]

But the 93rd performed so well in the battlefield and set exemplary standards of behavior, they were treated well by the French. Many wished to remain in France after the war because, for the first time, they experienced freedom and dignity. Despite receiving France's highest military award, the Croix de Guerre, as well as receiving more citations than any other AEF regiment, the black troops returned on segregated ships to an America that had not changed in its bias against blacks. W.E.B. DuBois wrote:

> But by the God of heaven, we are cowards and jackasses if now that the war is over, we do not marshal every ounce of our brain and brawn to fight a sterner, longer, more unbending battle against the forces of hell in our own land.
> We return.
> We return from fighting.
> We return fighting.
> Make way for Democracy! We saved it in France, and by the Great Jehovah, we will save it in the United States of America, or know the reason why.[29]

During World War I, several changes occurred that affected the African American's acceptance of society's concept that he was an inferior being and was supposed to be subservient to whites. Black soldiers were well received abroad and in some places, lived and worked together with whites. In the United States, the beginning of the industrialization of the South and the movement from the farm to the city led to the migration of blacks to the North. Returning veterans who had experienced what it meant to be free and to be treated with respect, refused to accept segregated drinking fountains, restaurants, and public transportation.

The soldiers resented the Jim Crow practices and focused their

Introduction

anger on the segregated streetcars, defying the seating restrictions and threatening to derail the cars. This resulted in repeated confrontations and on August 23, 1917, a member of the 24th Infantry stationed in Houston, Texas, came to the aid of a black woman who was being beaten by a white policeman. Although the officer's shots had missed the soldier, rumors spread at the fort that one of their troops had been killed by a racist cop. Two hundred soldiers disobeyed orders to stay on the base and raided the armory, where they took guns, heading to Houston. A shooting spree and fight resulted in the deaths of sixteen white civilians and four black soldiers. Following an investigation, fifty-four soldiers were court-martialed for mutiny and murder; forty-one were sentenced to life; and thirteen were condemned to hang.[30]

The consequences of the Houston mutiny and riot would influence the military in its assignment of black troops for years to come. The War Department no longer stationed large concentrations of black combat troops in the same military bases. Realizing that it was important to ensure the support of African Americans for the war against Germany, the army continued to enlist them, but made an effort to separate them from whites and to assign them to small units to minimize the possibility of protests and riots. Military leaders were also concerned about the loyalty of African Americans following the hangings of the Houston soldiers. This distrust and question of patriotism of blacks was later used by the Ku Klux Klan, who cited allegations by the black press of wartime mistreatment of black soldiers as proof of disloyalty.

The enactment of Selective Service legislation, instituting the military draft in 1917, led to a sharp increase in the number of black recruits. Because blacks were not represented on draft boards, they had little hope of avoiding military service unless they failed to meet the physical or mental standards. This presented a challenge to the War Department in their ability to absorb a large number in black recruits while maintaining segregated training and housing facilities. Following the violence in Houston, members of the General Staff issued a new policy making limited use of the blacks drafted through the selective service. The War Department would organize one black division, with only four infantry regiments and allow minimal training with

Introduction

weapons before shipping it overseas. All black draftees who were not assigned to this division would serve in noncombat units. Although draft legislation contained no specific racial provisions, local draft boards required black registrants to tear off one corner of their registration card so they could be more easily identified and inducted separately from whites.[31]

Believing that this laboring class of African Americans did not have the physical, mental, or moral character necessary to stand up to combat, military leaders assigned most of them to labor battalions. Comprising more than one-third of all labor troops, they constructed wharves, docks, railroads, and warehouses, repaired roads and loaded freight as well as buried fellow soldiers killed in action. Assigning blacks to labor units allowed more white troops to serve in the combat units, a policy rationalized by the War Department. This policy also prevented the training of large numbers of blacks in the use of firearms, lessoning the fears of many whites, especially Southerners.

The military's argument that colored troops could not be made efficient unless they had white officers was challenged in December 1917 by a committee of African American leaders led by Joel E. Spingarn, chairman of the Board of Directors of the National Association for the Advancement of Colored People (NAACP). The Wilson Administration and the army refused to integrate officer training camps, which would imply that there was equality between the races. Following continued pressure by African Americans in addition to the increasing need for additional troops, Secretary of War Baker proposed that the Army War College investigate the feasibility of training black junior officers to help lead the black units. The proposal was endorsed by the head of the War College Division of the General Staff, General Kuhn, with certain restrictions: "That colored officers should not be assigned to white organizations requires no argument, yet it is believed that there are many colored men of good character who, with training, would make suitable company officers for the colored organizations forming part of the contemplated drafted force."[32] An additional roadblock was contrived, for the proposal required Spingarn and his committee to obtain letters of intent from 200 college-educated men. The black collegiate community responded, providing more than 1500 names to the War Department.

Introduction

In June 1917, on orders of President Wilson, the army opened an officer training school for African Americans at Fort Des Moines, Iowa. There was a waiting list of 1200 educated African Americans from all parts of the country. The program graduated and commissioned 639 black officers before closing five months later.[33] Although the military had no official policy regarding the integration of African American officer candidates, the War Department announced that future candidates would attend regular officer training facilities. Each facility was allowed to determine its own policy, leaving some to continue to practice segregation. Over 700 additional African Americans graduated from these camps, bringing the total number of black officers serving in the war to 1353.[34] As the war progressed and the need for troops increased, black officers eventually began serving in hastily established service units that had become integrated. When the black officers joined a labor battalion, the white noncommissioned officers were transferred to units where they would be taking orders from officers of their own race. The idea that a black man could supervise whites was still unacceptable in the Jim Crow era. Black officers continued to experience discrimination, from the refusal of white enlisted men to salute them to being barred from officers' clubs and quarters.

Yet, despite the racial discrimination that existed among the troops, black leaders continued to rally young African Americans to enlist, after obtaining promises of improved racial conditions after the war by government officials. W.E.B. DuBois observed, "We of the colored race have no ordinary interest in the outcome, that which the German power represents today shall spell death to the aspirations of Negroes and all darker races for equality, freedom, and democracy. Let us not hesitate. Let us, while this war lasts, forget our special grievances and close ranks shoulder to shoulder with our own white fellow citizens and the allied nations that are fighting for democracy."[35]

When in 1918 the war ended, 6,000 African American soldiers had lost their lives in combat. But black veterans found that little had changed in the United State when it came to acceptance and equality for African Americans. Several veterans returning to the South were assaulted by white crowds at railway stations and stripped of their uniforms. That year, fifty-eight African Americans were lynched in the United States and seventy in 1919, many of them soldiers still in uni-

Introduction

form.[36] Black veterans were accused of being infected with "foreign ideas and by foreign women."

Many whites saw the increased efforts of the returning black troops for equal rights as a threat to maintaining African American subordination and, with the help of the Ku Klux Klan which had been dormant since the 1880s, renewed their reign of terror to suppress racial equality. Racial violence increased, resulting in the eruption of race riots in twenty-six cities across the country during the summer and fall of 1919.[37]

It would be many years before full integration and equal opportunity in the military would come for African Americans. Military policies were strongly influenced by the racial climate of American society and reflected the treatment of blacks in civilian life, but by demonstrating that large numbers of blacks and whites could live and work together, the military's experiences helped to shape the country's social policy.

1

Threats, Fear and Triumph
The Opening of the Tuskegee Veterans Hospital

ORDERS NEGRO DOCTORS TO TUSKEGEE HOSPITAL
    Director Himes, After Hearing Protests of Whites, Sustains the Former Decision
    WASHINGTON, Aug. 15.—After several conferences with white residents of Tuskegee, Ala. who have protested against the installation of negro personnel at the veterans' hospital there, Director Hines of the veterans' hospital has selected six negro physicians for duty in the institution and expects them to leave for their post within the next week or ten days.—*New York Times*, August 16, 1923

The assignment of the six black doctors to the United States Veterans Hospital in Tuskegee that August marked the end of a year-long struggle that was embedded in the refusal of the Veterans Bureau to replace the hospital's all-white medical staff with black health care professionals. Four of the young men, George Branche, Harvey Davis, Simon O. Johnson, and Toussaint Tilton, shared a common bond: graduates of prominent Boston medical schools, they had also been trained by Dr. Solomon Carter Fuller, America's first African American psychiatrist and a renowned neuropathologist.

The events leading up to this historical occasion began in March 1921 when the Consultants on Hospitalization were appointed by Secretary of the Treasury Andrew Mellon to advise him on the development of a national hospital system for veterans. The consultants were known as the White Committee, named for its chairperson, Dr. William Charles White, a Pittsburgh physician who was an expert in both psychiatry and tuberculosis. For two years, with the assistance of an

The Tuskegee Veterans Hospital and Its Black Physicians

advisory group that included members of the United States Public Health Service, the National Committee for Mental Hygiene, the National Home for Disabled Volunteer Soldiers, and the National Tuberculosis Association, the committee collected and analyzed data on the number of veterans and their medical needs as well as the number of hospitals that would be required to care for them.[1] Although the legislation that mandated the Veterans Bureau to establish hospitals throughout the country had not addressed the issue of separate facilities for black veterans, the White Committee found that little effort was being made to treat the 400,000 African Americans who served the United States in World War I.[2]

Before World War I, few hospitals existed in the United States specifically for the care of African Americans and most medical facilities in the South refused to treat them. Barred from most hospitals, many disabled black veterans were being sent to private hospitals that provided poor care, were housed in jails or mental institutions or, frequently, were not receiving care at all even though seriously disabled. Those who were able to gain admission to predominately white hospitals were placed in segregated wards where they received inferior care. Approximately 300,000 of the African Americans who served in the war were natives of the Southern states. For those black soldiers who lived in the South, it was almost impossible to obtain treatment.[3]

In June 1921, a decision was reached by the White Committee, without any input from black organizations, to address the so-called "Negro problem" by recommending a separate health care facility in the South for the black soldier. With Alabama and Georgia having the largest numbers of black soldiers who were veterans of World War I (40 percent each), they became the prime contenders for the location of the hospital.

Despite considerable resistance from the area's white population, Secretary Mellon approved $2,250,000 for the construction of a 500-bed hospital at Tuskegee, Alabama, on November 18, 1921.

> To the honorable the Secretary of the Treasury, Washington
>
> Sir: Your consultants on hospitalization beg to recommend an allotment of $2,250,000 for the provision of a hospital for tuberculosis and nervous and mental cases among the negro ex-service men.

1. Threats, Fear and Triumph

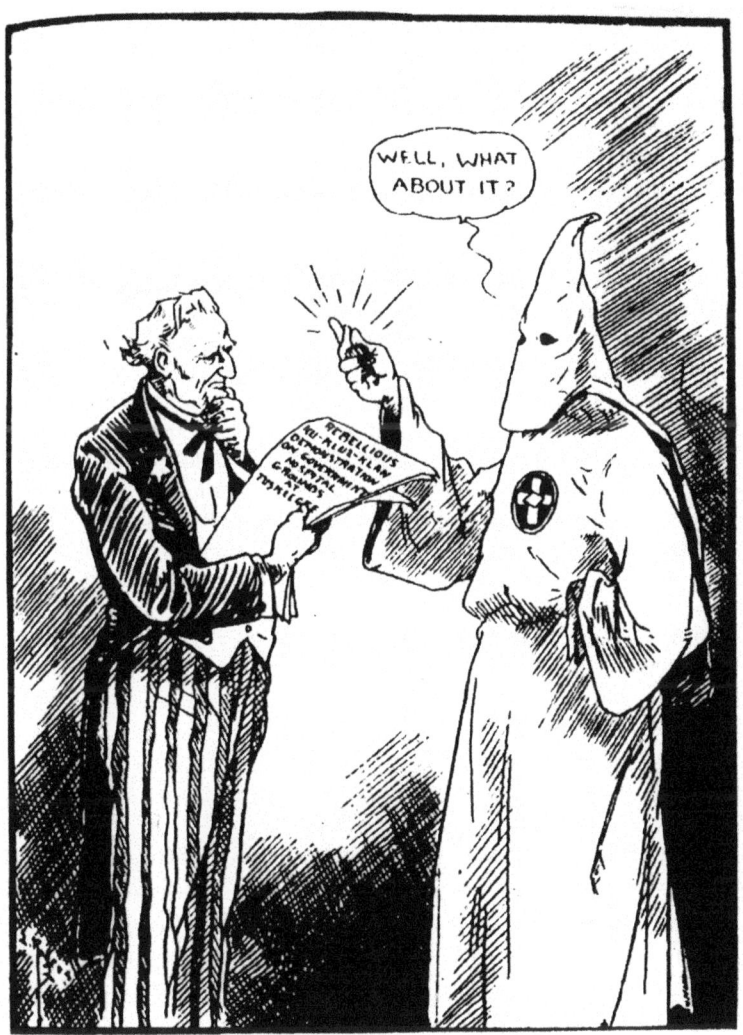

Editorial cartoon, criticizing government position on Tuskegee Veterans Hospital, *Chicago Defender,* **July 21, 1923.**

The sum here allotted will be used for the following:

For neuropsychiatric patients. Standard units previously approved by your board of consultants to accommodate 230 patients of this class; also the buildings for utilities, such as mess hall and kitchen, etc.

For tuberculosis patients. There would be included one wing of the infirmary

The Tuskegee Veterans Hospital and Its Black Physicians

according to the standard approved type and units for semi ambulant and ambulant patients to bring accommodations for tuberculosis patients up to the number of 270, making a total for all patients of 500.

There would also be constructed a general administration building, recreation building, and general utility buildings, such as power house, laundry, storage buildings, garage, quarters for personnel, etc. There would be further included expenditures for water supply, roads, and other items of outside service.

The plan upon which this hospital is being constructed contemplates its enlargement to 1,000 beds. The cost per bed, therefore, is greater than that necessary for the number of beds here described. A fair percentage of the utilities here provided should fittingly be charged to the cost of future beds to be provided.

The hospital is to be placed upon the site donated to the United States Government by the board of trustees of the Tuskegee Normal and Industrial Institute. The purchase of certain tracts of ground for the protection of this site is included in appropriation. The provision of a spur of railroad from the Western Railroad of Alabama, approximately 1¾ miles to this site, has already been arranged for. The final plans, specifications, and details in connection with the utilities and purchase will come before the consultants for final approval.

Respectfully submitted.
William Charles White, Chairman.
Frank Billings
John G. Bowman
George H. Kirby
Consultants on Hospitalization.
Approved November 16, 1921.—W. Mellon[4]

Fears about the neuropsychiatric and tuberculosis patients who would be treated at the hospital as well as resistance to the plans to eventually staff the hospital with black personnel resulted in heightened racial tensions, with white Tuskegeeans seeing the hospital as danger to the community and a challenge to the supremacy of the Anglo-Saxon race. A letter to the *Montgomery Advertiser* stated, "When the Government agents were trying to find a place suitable for the Negro veterans' hospital, they came to Montgomery. Our people did not want it.... The Northern Negro wouldn't have good health in the Southern climate; nothing here would make him happy; and certainly he doesn't suit our people.... Our people will not stand for it."[5]

The NAACP and a national committee of black veterans were also opposed to locating the facility in the South. The NAACP contended

1. Threats, Fear and Triumph

that black veterans should receive treatment in the same hospitals as white veterans. They also thought that by placing black veterans in the heart of the segregated South, they would be subjected to inferior treatment. W.E.B. DuBois observed, "Black soldiers should be cared for without discrimination in the same hospitals and under the same circumstances as white soldiers. But even if this were impossible because of race hatred, certainly the last place on God's green earth to put a segregated Negro hospital was in the lynching-belt of mob-ridden Alabama, Georgia, Mississippi and their ilk ... there is no protection in central Alabama for a decent Negro pig-pen, much less for an institution to restore the life and health of those very black servants of the nation."[6] Walter White, assistant secretary of the NAACP, believed, "The gathering together of any considerable number of colored ex-soldiers, even though they be invalids, would cause opposition in the South. The South does not want any [black] men who have learned how to fight."[7]

Several members of the National Committee of Negro Veteran Relief, an organization founded by veterans of the world war to ensure that they would receive the benefits owed them under the Veterans Bureau legislation, met with William Charles White on November 1, 1921, to voice their opposition to the construction of the hospital in the South.[8] In the seven months that the Consultants on Hospitalization had solicited information and heard testimony about the proposed black veterans hospital, the National Committee of Negro Veteran Relief had never been contacted. When Lieutenant John W. Love, chairperson of the committee, learned of the proposed hospital through the press, he requested a meeting with White, who claimed that he had no knowledge of the organization. Fearing that locating the hospital in the South would further segregation, the Committee contended that instead of admitting Northern black veterans to hospitals in their areas, they would all be transported to the black veterans hospital in the South. They recommended that the hospital be located in Washington, D.C., near Howard University, arguing that the Tuskegee location was not near a large medical center. White defended the decision of the Consultants on Hospitalization to locate the hospital in Tuskegee, maintaining that locating it in the South was not an attempt to segregate, but to provide better care to Southern veterans. While he

The Tuskegee Veterans Hospital and Its Black Physicians

reassured the Committee that veterans hospitals in the North would admit African Americans, he did not guarantee that they would not be placed in segregated wards.

A black organization that was surprisingly absent from the debate was the National Medical Association. Despite the fact that the editor of the *Journal of the National Medical Association*, Dr. John A. Kenney, was the medical director at Tuskegee Institute's John A. Andrew Memorial Hospital, there was no attempt by the organization to provide input to the White Committee. There was only one letter on record sent to White on November 18, 1921 (two days following the approval of the construction of the hospital at Tuskegee) from Dr. J. A. Lester, secretary of association's commission on medical education, recommending that the hospital be built in Nashville near Meharry Medical College.

A deciding factor to locate the hospital in Tuskegee was the offer by Tuskegee Institute to donate 300 of the 464 acres needed to the government for construction of the hospital buildings. The mayor of Tuskegee, William Varner, considering the possible economic benefits of locating the hospital in the area, had urged Dr. Robert Moton, president of the Tuskegee Institute, to use his influence with President Harding. In addition to the donation of a portion of the school's land, Mayor Varner also made it known that he had adjacent property available for the VA to purchase.

Tuskegee had already established a hospital in 1893 on its campus to care for the school's faculty and students. What was originally the student infirmary, the John A. Andrew Memorial Hospital had expanded to serve the health needs of local African American residents, neighboring communities, and, eventually, out-of-state patients. Under its director, Dr. John A. Kenney, the hospital established a training school for black nurses and operated a vocational rehabilitation program for black veterans. Beginning in 1912, the hospital was the site of the National Medical Association's annual meeting held each April to coincide with Negro Health Week. In conjunction with the professional meeting, a clinic was held to treat blacks in the area who were unable to pay for health care. Over the years, the clinic became a centerpiece of promoting public health for African Americans, with people arriving two days in advance for the three-day clinic where they were treated

1. Threats, Fear and Triumph

for free by physicians and surgeons from throughout the region who would donate their services.[9]

The college agreed to house the black employees who would eventually join the hospital staff, and Dr. Robert R. Moton and its Board of Trustees promised to use their influence with the white citizens of Tuskegee as well as the state of Alabama to obtain their support of a black staff. Members of the White Committee considered the school, which was established by Booker T. Washington in 1881, to be the center of African American learning in the country and its president a respected advisor to several white politicians and philanthropists on racial issues. George Washington Carver, the head of the school's agricultural program and director of the country's only black agricultural experiment station, had also gained the respect of "white" Tuskegee as a highly regarded scientist. It was not unusual for Institute faculty to socialize with some of the prominent white Tuskegee citizens, although the black visitors were careful to enter their homes through the back door. Whites were welcomed to religious and cultural events at the school, which provided a separate seating area for them near the front of the chapel.[10] According to the Report of the Consultants on Hospitalization, "The question of the location of such an institution was more difficult than had been foreseen. The objections of communities, the personal interests of various bodies, and the views of experts made a problem of great complexity. Accepting, however, as an axiom that the more satisfactory solution rested largely with the colored people themselves, it was finally decided that the location of such an institution in the center of negro education, conducted under negro leadership, would probably bring about the best results."[11]

The practice of blacks serving in the military under white commanders was to be carried over into the new VA hospital. While the Treasury Department's hospitalization committee did agree to have black physicians on the Tuskegee hospital staff, it made the point that the hospital would be under the management of white physicians who had experience in the treatment of the diseases for which the hospital was established. So willing to maintain an amicable relationship with the federal government as well the local white citizens, Dr. Moton did not object when the decision was made to place the hospital under the operation and control of white administrators who understood the

The Tuskegee Veterans Hospital and Its Black Physicians

Southern point of view on race relations. Moton believed that without the promise of white management of the hospital, the leading citizens of Tuskegee would have opposed it and the hospital would not have been built in the town. The dominant white society accepted irresponsibility, ignorance and submissiveness as typical traits of the Negro. Those blacks who did not fit the stereotype were seen as deviant and to be feared. Frederick Douglass stated, "The resistance is not to the colored man as a slave, a servant or a menial. It is aimed at the Negro as a man.... It is only when he acquires education, property, and influence, only when he attempts to rise and be a man among men that he invites repression. It is not to the Negro but the quality in which he comes which makes him an offense."[12] Leon Litwack put it this way: "There was one thing that the white South feared more than Negro dishonesty, ignorance and incompetency, and that was Negro honesty, knowledge and efficiency."[13]

In May 1922, the $1,010,000 building contract was awarded to the Algernon Blair Construction Company of Montgomery, Alabama.[14] Initially the hospital plans called for twenty-seven buildings, with a capacity of 500 beds, the majority housing neuropsychiatric patients. Other beds were to be used for patients with tuberculosis and venereal disease, medical conditions commonly thought to be essentially Negro problems, as well as general medical, surgical, and neurological illnesses.

As construction on the new hospital began in the summer of 1922, there was increasing pressure from the black community for the government to appoint blacks to the professional staff. After meeting with Moton that June, Colonel Charles F. Forbes, director of the Veterans Bureau, ordered that preparations begin to build a staff of black professionals to run the new facility.[15, 16] As the building project neared completion, Moton asked Melvin J. Chisum, the field secretary of the National Negro Press Association and a Washington contact for the Tuskegee Institute, to check on the progress of staff recruitment. Assured by the Veterans Bureau that plans were underway to hire black professionals, Chisum found that this was not in fact true. While visiting the St. Paul, Minnesota, veterans hospital, shortly before the Tuskegee hospital was scheduled to open, he came upon a notice posted in the main lobby announcing the availability of positions at "the new U.S. Veterans Hospital for colored veterans at Tuskegee."

1. Threats, Fear and Triumph

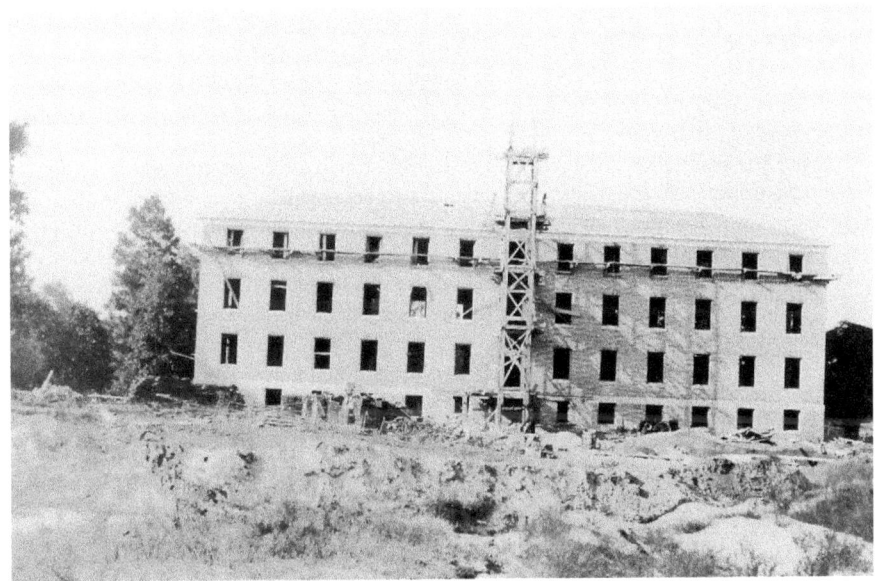

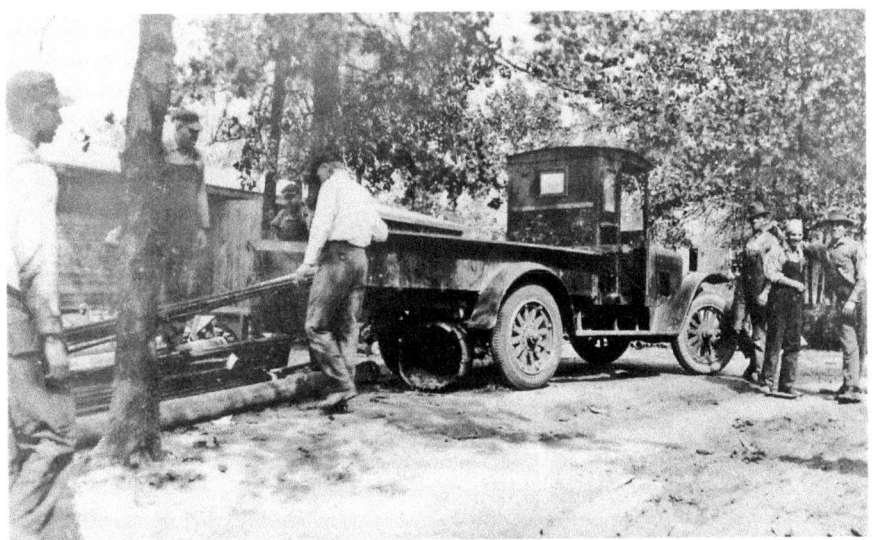

Top: Construction of the Tuskegee Veterans Hospital, 1922. *Bottom:* Black and white laborers at the construction of the Tuskegee Veterans Hospital, 1922 (Tuskegee University Archives, Tuskegee, Alabama).

The Tuskegee Veterans Hospital and Its Black Physicians

> The new U.S. Veterans Hospital for Colored Veterans at Tuskegee, Alabama, the finest of its kind in the world, is being constructed by the U.S. Treasury Department, and will probably be completed between February 10 and 25. The sum allotted for the construction of this hospital by the Treasury Department was $2,250,000.
>
> The plans allow for about 600 beds—302 tuberculosis patients and 294 for neuropsychiatric patients. The medical personnel will be composed of white persons. The chief nurse, chief aides, chief dietitian, and their assistants will be white. The staff nurse, aides and dietitians will probably be colored. The medical coordinator selected to take charge of this hospital will be from the Reserve Corps of the Public Health Service, of Southern birth, and one who thoroughly understands the Negro.
>
> The colored people of Tuskegee and the superintendent and staff of Tuskegee Institute are giving Government officials their hearty cooperation.[17]

The exclusion of blacks in the operation of the hospital was not limited to hospital staff positions. The contract for burying the soldiers who expired in the hospital was given to a white undertaker from Greenville, South Carolina, before the bids of local black undertakers had a chance to be submitted.[18]

Veterans Hospital Number 91 for Negro Disabled Soldiers opened on February 12, 1923. The significance of choosing Lincoln's birthday to open the first government hospital to treat black veterans was not lost on Vice President Calvin Coolidge, who came to make the dedication speech in the Chapel of Tuskegee Institute. In part, he said:

> For the service of the Negro race at home and abroad during the war, they have the everlasting gratitude of America. They have justified Abraham Lincoln.... It is well for us, who must live together as Americans, whatever our race or creed may be, constantly to remember the words of Lincoln: "We are not enemies, but friends. We must not be enemies." Those who stir up animosities, those who create any kind of hatred and enmity are not ministering to the public welfare. We have come out of a war with a desire and a determination to live at peace with the world. Out of a common suffering and a common sacrifice there came a new meaning to our common citizenship. Our greatest need is to live in harmony, in friendship and in good will, not seeking an advantage over each other, but all trying to serve each other. In that spirit let us dedicate this hospital and dedicate ourselves to the service of our country. To do that wisely, patiently, tolerantly, is to show by the discharge of our duties our indisputable title to fellow citizenship with Lincoln.[19]

Other dignitaries on the dedication platform included Alabama governor William W. Brandon, commander of the Alabama Division

The Tuskegee Student

VOL. 33 MARCH 1-15, 1923 Nos. 5-6

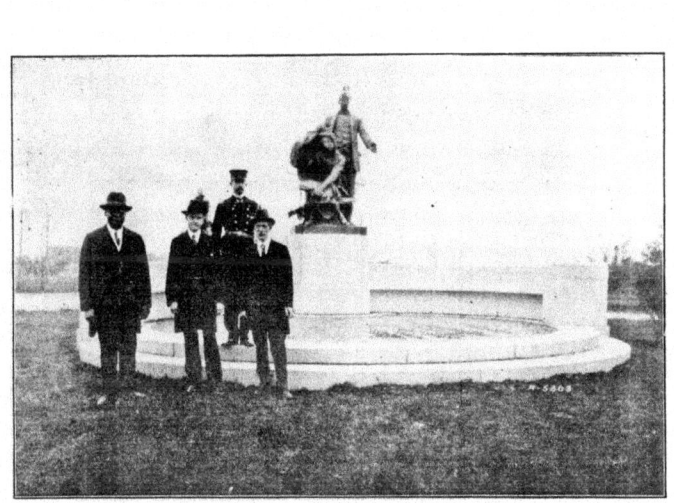

PRINCIPAL SPEAKERS AT THE DEDICATION
OF GOVERNMENT HOSPITAL

Dr. Robert R. Moton, Principal of Tuskegee Institute, the
Hon. Calvin Coolidge, Vice-president of the United States,
the Hon. W. W. Brandon, Governor of Alabama and
Captain S. S. Yeandel, Aide to the Vice-president in
front of the Booker T. Washington Memorial

Cover of *The Tuskegee Student*, March 1–15, 1923, Vol. 33, Nos. 5–6 (Tuskegee University Archives, Tuskegee, Alabama).

of the American Legion, General Robert E. Steiner, Dr. W. E. White of the United States Treasury Department, and assistant secretary of the treasury, Colonel E. Clifford. Representing the Institute and the African American community, Dr. Moton spoke of the efforts made by his predecessor, Booker T. Washington, to establish at Tuskegee a platform where black and white men could discuss the difficulties which they faced in common and make plans to work together. He pledged the Institute's support of the hospital, stating the hospital "marks the greatest physical achievement of our government for the Negro race in America since Emancipation." Roger E. Macdonald, a disabled black soldier who was being rehabilitated at Tuskegee Institute, spoke for the African American veterans. "It was a marvelous thing for the Negro race, itself so long oppressed, to have an opportunity to help save others from oppression, and let it be said to the eternal credit of the Negro soldiers that they made good that opportunity."[20]

Suspended over the speaker's platform next to the American flag was a service flag in honor of the 600 Tuskegee citizens who served in the recent war. The chapel was filled to capacity that afternoon, with many having to stand outside to hear the speeches and the music sung by the Tuskegee Institute Choir. The choir sang several spirituals and the audience clamored for more. As the choir began singing "Let Us Cheer the Weary Traveler," Colonel Clifford noticed that the vice president appeared disinterested, and concerned that he was growing weary of the music, leaned over and whispered, "If you are tired of the singing I will stop it and go ahead with the program." Without taking his eyes away from choir, Mr. Coolidge whispered, "I like it."[21]

The festivities began earlier that morning when the vice-president and his party arrived and went immediately to inspect the twenty-seven buildings of the hospital. Following the inspection, the party went to the Institute, where they were welcomed by Dr. Moton and 2000 teachers and students. A luncheon and tour of the Institute were provided and the vice president then reviewed the Reserve Officers' Training Corps, which was under the command of Lieutenant Colonel B. O. Davis, the highest ranking Negro officer in the U.S. army.

The final cost of the hospital, which was now the third largest veterans hospital and the most significant federal project built for African Americans, came to more than $2,500,000.

Despite the Veterans Bureau order for the hospital to be run by a black staff, the facility opened with an all-white staff and a white Alabamian, Colonel Robert H. Stanley, as the chief medical officer in charge.[22] A press release from the Veterans Bureau announced that

1. Threats, Fear and Triumph

"the medical officer selected to take charge of this hospital will be from the Reserve Corps of the Public Health Service, of southern birth, and one who thoroughly understands the Negro."[23] According to a report by the NAACP, "A Major Kenzie was sent to Tuskegee and he, in sounding out local White People, promised them unconditionally that the hospital would be manned by an entire white staff. Before Major Moton and his associates knew of the plans, Colonel Robert H. Stanley, a southern white man who is a vicious hater of Negroes, had assumed charge of the hospital."[24]

The colonel, a childhood friend of General Steiner, had opposed the construction of a black veterans hospital in Montgomery. In the months preceding Colonel Stanley's appointment, the Veterans Bureau had persistently evaded Dr. Moton's questions about what their personnel policy would be and he was told that the "right type of man" would be appointed and that Moton would be consulted before the appointment was made. In spite of the bureau's promise to keep him informed, Stanley had been appointed superintendent of the hospital and was in Tuskegee for two days before Moton learned of the appointment.[25]

Even though the hospital was to provide care for black veterans, it was thought that there was not a sufficient number of competent, well-trained black health care professionals to run it. Stanley rejected Moton's recommendation that at least a small number of black physicians and nurses be hired, considering it a violation of Jim Crow racial segregation. Moton's suggestion that Dr. John A. Kenney, the medical director and chief surgeon at the John A. Andrew Memorial Hospital on the Tuskegee Institute campus, be appointed at the veterans hospital as a consultant, was also dismissed by Stanley, who stated that such proposals were not to be taken seriously. He wrote to President Moton:

> It was deemed wise by the Veterans Bureau to place white officers in charge and a man of your perspicuity must fully appreciate the fact that it would be utterly impossible to function successfully with a mixed staff of white and colored officers. For the same reasons, it is equally impossible to function with white officers and negro consultants. I can but believe that the recommendation that negro officers be put on the staff was made for diplomatic reasons alone. A man of your mental ability and your knowledge of the situation would no more approve such a mixture than I would.[26]

The Tuskegee Veterans Hospital and Its Black Physicians

The only concession made by Stanley to integrating the hospital staff was the hiring of black nurse aides, orderlies, attendants, and laborers. Under the Health Care Segregation Law, passed in 1915 in Alabama, it was illegal for white women to be forced to care for black men, so a black nurse-maid was assigned to each white nurse. The law provided that "no person or corporation shall require any white female nurse in wards or rooms in hospitals, either public or private, in which Negro men are placed."[27]

The person considered to be the instigator of efforts to bar black professionals from the hospital staff was Major George E. Ijams, the acting director of the Veterans Bureau who had appointed Stanley. Ijams informed the White House that he only hired white personnel at Tuskegee after failing to find black professionals who met Civil Service eligibility standards. Strong resistance to having blacks join the hospital staff also came from General Robert E. Steiner, head of Alabama's American Legion. General Steiner had fought the proposal made at the organization's national meeting to admit Negro veterans to membership. As a consequence of the defeat of the proposal, those veterans had no affiliation with the American Legion and were not given any recognition by the Alabama chapter.

Moton went to see the president, Warren G. Harding, informing him of Stanley's betrayal of the original agreement and warning him of the repercussions coming from the black press and black voters, many of whom were loyal supporters of the Republican Party. Responding to the pleas urging that blacks be considered for positions on the hospital's medical staff by Moton and by James Weldon Johnson, secretary of the NAACP, President Harding issued a directive on February 23: "There should be no designation of officials and nurses for the care of the colored soldiers at the United States Veterans Hospital at Tuskegee until there has been a thorough and determined effort to secure a civil service eligible list of colored citizens."[28]

The task of recruiting black physicians was a formidable one and the Veterans Bureau enlisted the help of Moton, Dr. Michael O. Dumas of the National Medical Association (NMA), and the NAACP.[29] Originally, the NMA had opposed the location of the hospital in Tuskegee because of the concern that it would lead to the establishment of a medical school that would take funds and prestige away from the other

1. Threats, Fear and Triumph

established black medical schools. Advised by Moton of the difficulty in qualifying blacks for professional positions due to the inability of the Civil Service Commission to identify the race of applicants, Harding issued an executive order authorizing special examinations for Negro applicants. These examinations were advertised in the Negro press and by the National Medical Association. Fifteen thousand copies of the examination announcement were distributed to black institutions and to 250 black publications.[30] In May, it was reported that forty black nurses had passed the examinations and were to be placed at Tuskegee and that when qualified black physicians were found, they would also be sent. Hines also announced plans to visit the hospital, at which time he would announce the selection of the "colored surgeon-in-chief who will have charge of the hospital."

Not surprisingly, a storm of protest against placing the hospital under the control of black staff irrupted from white Alabamians. U.S. Senator Thomas Heflin said, "Ordinarily, I would say that it is all right for a negro hospital to be operated in every way by negroes.... I was convinced that there was a distinct understanding between the government at Washington and the white people of Tuskegee that if they would consent for the negro hospital to be located there that it should be under control of white officials." State Senator R.H. Powell added, "We do not want any Government institution in Alabama with niggers in charge. White supremacy in this state must be maintained at any cost and we are not going to have any niggers in the state whom we cannot control." Albion Hosley, in a letter to John Calhoun, wrote, "The hospital here is the very best of the Hospitals which have been erected by the Government. The Officers Quarters and the Nurses Quarters are most beautifully equipped and appointed, and it is this situation which is a source of irritation to the Southern whites. They are determined to keep Negroes from holding important positions here, if they can prevent it."[31]

Prominent white Alabamians also argued that exclusively white operation of the hospital would have a significant financial impact on the town. The economic prosperity created by the construction workers who built the hospital would suffer with only black personnel and patients, who could not spend money at local businesses that excluded black people. "The truth of the matter is that the whites are making a desperate effort to hold on to the Tuskegee Hospital because when it is fully staffed there will be payroll of $75,000 per month, and it is this money which they want to get into the hands of white people."[32]

With pressure from white elected officials as well as citizens from Alabama, the president, who while not refusing to change his directive, reneged on his promise to have black staff hired in time for the opening of the hospital and told a group of black politicians that the "time was not ripe" for black personnel.[33] Despite the reassurance by Helen H. Gardner of the Civil Service Commission that there were qualified black physicians available in the specialties needed at Tuskegee, Hines told George E. Cannon of the National Medical Association that due to difficulties in finding black physicians who were specialists in treating tuberculosis and neuropsychiatric disorders he had decided to open the hospital with a white physician staff.

With indications that the Harding Administration had begun to retreat from its position, a white citizens' committee turned their efforts to putting pressure on Dr. Moton to accept white control of the hospital. Several anonymous threats were made against his life, resulting in guards being stationed on the Tuskegee Institute campus as well as at his home, and his family being sent to their summer home at Cappahosic, Virginia. Fifteen white citizens of the community came to Moton's office with a petition and demanded that he sign a statement supporting white management of the hospital or risk the destruction of Tuskegee Institute. Part of the petition said: "Booker Washington gave thirty-five years of his life to build up this school. You, unless you are too stubborn to sign a little paper here, are going to have it all blown up in twenty-four hours.... You understand that we have the legislation, we make the laws, we have the judges, the sheriffs, the jails. We have the hardware stores and the arms.... A thousand men—their spokesman called me up this morning—will be over on an hour's notice and wipe out the whole institution if things are not going the way we want them to go.... Your life is in our hands."[34]

Moton, who had tried to compromise in the past, refused to yield to white racism and replied:

> All my life.... I have believed that white and colored Southerners could work together. If I am mistaken in this view, then the best thing that can happen to me is to die. You say my life is in your hands. I do not doubt it. You have in

1. Threats, Fear and Triumph

your hands all the things you have mentioned—the laws, the judges, the jails and even the guns.... I haven't a gun in my pocket or anywhere else.... You can wipe me out, you can take my life, gentlemen, but you can't take my character. If Negroes who are thoroughly educated and trained for such service can't serve their own people, can't serve in that hospital, on land given by a Negro school, for Negro veterans, provided by the Federal Government, if they can't practice in that hospital, then you may as well wipe out Tuskegee Institute and every other Negro institution in the world. The sooner you do it the better. If I were to sign that paper, I would be deceiving my people and country. It's a Negro hospital built for Negroes; and gentlemen, if Negroes trained for the job can't run it, you can wipe out the hospital and the school and Moton.[35]

President Moton, realizing that by taking his stand against the white committeemen, his life was in danger and that he could not continue this fight on his own, enlisted the help of the NAACP. Under the association's direction, a campaign was waged through the press and by telegrams to government officials. Editorials were submitted that focused on the hypocrisy of segregationists and white supremacists who argued that the hospital should be staffed by white employees whose jobs would be to serve and wait upon black patients. Letters were written to the editors of several newspapers, suggesting that whites were only interested in the hospital's payroll. The *Atlanta Independent* published an editorial on May 24, 1923, charging that

> the white man has not given a single reason why he should be put in charge of the hospital at Tuskegee, and our group can see but one reason why he wants it and that is to satisfy his lust for power and greed for money. It is not that he loves the Negro so well that he wants him to have the very best services that man is capable of rendering. He wants to boss, he wants to control; he wants to keep the Negro down and shut him out from every opportunity that will enable him to measure up as a man. It is money and power the white man wants, and not service to black men.[36]

The economic incentive to maintain white control of the hospital was also emphasized by W. E. B. Dubois: "The only interest of white people in Alabama in this hospital is economic and racial. They want to draw the government salaries and they do not want any Negro officials in Alabama whom the State cannot dominate."[37]

As the controversy continued to escalate, guards were placed around Moton's house. The NNACP, fearing violence, asked President Harding to send federal troops to Tuskegee to protect Moton and the

The Tuskegee Veterans Hospital and Its Black Physicians

college campus. Moton was advised to remove himself from the increasingly dangerous controversy and in June, he left Tuskegee for three months to work with government officials in Washington. Booker T. Washington's widow, Margaret, and Dr. John A. Kenney, a prominent black physician in Tuskegee and a potential candidate to head the new hospital, fearing for their safety, also left the area. The personal physician to both George Washington Carver and Booker T. Washington and an outspoken advocate for black professional staff at the Tuskegee hospital, Dr. Kenney and his family fled the town after the Ku Klux Klan burned a cross on his lawn and threatened his life. Dr. Kenny went to the home of Dr. George Cannon, chairman of the executive board of the National Medical Association, who organized a committee to bring the issue of a Negro staff at the hospital to the federal government's attention, resulting in several conferences being held with President Harding and General Hines.

Despite government assurances that the Tuskegee Veterans Hospital would be staffed by Negro employees and the growing numbers of white Southerners who believed that black doctors and nurses should provide care for disabled black veterans, when the hospital officially admitted its first patients on May 20, 1923, the professional staff was still entirely white. The black nurse-maids who provided basic daily care to the patients were paid $50 a month, while the white nurses received civil service salaries that ranged from $1680 to $2500 a year. The Veterans Bureau insisted that this situation was temporary and would change as soon as the Civil Service Commission could provide lists of a sufficient number of eligible black personnel to meet the needs of the hospital.[38] But Melvin Chisum had learned that the Veterans Bureau, where many departments were headed by white Southerners, was, in fact, conspiring "to defeat President Harding's and Moton's plan of staffing the Tuskegee Hospital with colored professionals."[39]

There were many in the Veterans Bureau who believed that there were few blacks available who were competent to run a large government hospital. Dr. Moton related an incident in which he challenged this assumption by the acting director of the bureau, Major George Ijams. When asked if there were any hospitals which offered training for Negro doctors and nurses, Dr. Moton replied, "Right here in Washington there is the Medical School of Howard University for training

1. Threats, Fear and Triumph

Negro physicians and the Freedman's Hospital and Nurse Training School, both supported by the government."[40] Expressing surprise, Ijams said that he had never heard of Howard University, the Freedman's Hospital or the National Medical Association, which had a membership of more than 3000 black physicians. Led by Ijams, a report was issued that contended that there were no Negroes capable of holding staff positions at the hospital and it was learned that the Veterans Bureau had rejected more than 50 applications from black physicians and nurses. For some job categories such as dieticians, there were no black applicants to be found due to the racial barriers that existed in those professions. Despite the challenges, efforts continued to recruit black personnel. The assistant director of the Veterans Bureau, L. B. Rogers, worked with the National Medical Association to obtain a list of qualified black physicians and identified thirty-three who had met the civil service eligibility requirements. For many black health care professionals who met the qualifications, persuading them to accept a position in a Southern town where racism was common and the potential for racial violence was a daily threat was a difficult sell.

By June 30, 1923, there were thirteen patients and 176 personnel at the Tuskegee hospital.[41] Among the personnel were five black nurses who had been hired earlier that month. Brigadier General Frank T. Hines, the newly appointed director of the Veterans Bureau, soon realized that a system of discrimination was in place to prevent blacks from qualifying for staff positions and assumed personal responsibility for finding qualified black professionals. Hines found that some black politicians were using the demand for black professionals as a pretense to use the hospital for patronage appointments. He was alerted by Moton and the NAACP that two prominent black politicians who were members of the Republican National Committee, Perry Howard from Mississippi and Henry Lincoln "Line" Johnson from Georgia, were attempting to have the Civil Service examinations waived in order to place their own men at Tuskegee to take control of the hospital's payroll and supplies. Hines admonished the politicians and issued a public letter reaffirming the administration's commitment to a black staff, but also stating that "it is not the intention of the bureau to man the hospital by a complete colored personnel."[42] Fearing that the sudden intrusion of large numbers of black professionals would trigger racial violence

The Tuskegee Veterans Hospital and Its Black Physicians

in Tuskegee, Hines announced on June 26 that the Veterans Bureau would temporarily halt the recruitment of black personnel, and with Moton's approval he decided to proceed to gradually introduce black professionals while maintaining white leadership of the hospital. But the white Southerners continued to press for a confrontation, arguing that black physicians and soldiers, many of whom had lived in the North and in other countries where they were accustomed to more freedom, would challenge the Southern tradition of white supremacy and black subordination. Adding to their fears was the belief that many of the black veterans were "shell-shocked and many of them mentally unbalanced" and that "it would be impossible to prevent bootleggers and dope vendors from selling their wares to them and that when these disabled veterans became charged with bad liquor and dope a colored staff would be unable to control them."[43] Alabama state senator Richard Holmes Powell contended, "We of the South ... know the Negro far better than the Northerner does. We know that the Negro cannot control even himself. The white race is the controlling race. Here in Tuskegee, our ratio is about one [white] to four and a half [blacks]. Here the white man has controlled and will continue to control."[44]

Despite Hines' plan to ease the racial tension surrounding the hiring of hospital staff by proceeding slowly, the situation escalated with the arrival of the hospital's first black professional on July 3, 1923. John H. Calhoun, a graduate of Hampton Institute, had passed the Civil Service examination for chief accountant, making the highest grade, while Clara Hunicutt, the white woman who had been temporarily appointed to the position, failed the exam. Mr. Calhoun arrived at the hospital to find that he had been given a desk but no assignment and was met at the door by Colonel Robert H. Stanley, the medical officer in charge, who gave orders that Calhoun was to be escorted out of the hospital by three armed white guards, and handed him a letter in a sealed envelope, which had no postmark or stamp. Fearing for his safety, Calhoun left the hospital and went to stay at Tuskegee Institute.

On the day of John Calhoun's arrival at the VA hospital, the Ku Klux Klan held a rally in Montgomery, the state capital. Following the rally, high ranking Klansmen were transported in a seventy-car caravan to Tuskegee, where at the railroad station they were met by several

1. Threats, Fear and Triumph

hundred members. Led by a large car displaying a massive American flag, the white supremacists marched through the town in a single file that covered more than two miles. Black residents had been advised to stay in their homes with their lights out during the demonstration in order to avoid violence. In the darkness, the hooded group burned a forty-foot cross outside of town and then, in silence, continued their march past Tuskegee Institute to the hospital. The Klan's decision to bypass the campus may have been influenced by the news that graduates and friends of the Institute had arrived that same afternoon from Montgomery, Birmingham, and Mobile, armed and outraged that Booker T. Washington's school was being threatened. The commander of the Tuskegee Institute Cadet Corps, Colonel William H. Walcott, stationed the school's protectors around the buildings and across the access routes. When the march ended, it was reported that twenty of the Klan demonstrators who were employees of the hospital disrobed in the woods near the hospital and returned to the facility. It was rumored that those employees were admitted to the government property by hospital security, searched it for John Calhoun, and were served a midnight meal prepared by the chief dietician.[45]

Following an investigation by the NNACP, charges were made against Colonel Stanley for additional activities that took place during the Klan march as well as for other acts of discrimination. According to a NAACP press release, these charges included:

1. That ten sheets from the storeroom of the Tuskegee Veterans Hospital were used in the Ku Klux Klan parade held on July 3 to terrorize colored personnel sent to work at the hospital by the Veterans Bureau. There was dust, automobile grease and other evidence to show the use to which the sheets had been put.
2. That on the evening of the parade, all of the white personnel left the Hospital with the exception of a few guards and that after the parade a group of twenty Klansmen came to the Hospital. The guards saluted these masked men and permitted them to search several of the building for John H. Calhoun, a Colored man whose life had been threatened that day by the Klan.

The Tuskegee Veterans Hospital and Its Black Physicians

3. As an instance of the discrimination practiced against colored people, for whose use the Hospital was built, the following order was signed by Col. Stanley: "U.S. Veterans Hospital No. 91, Tuskegee, Alabama, July 10, 1923, Hospital Order No. 15, giving the bus schedule is hereby amended for Sundays only, as follows: The bus that has been leaving at 10 A.M. is discontinued. The bus will leave the Hospital at 9:30 A.M. and returning will leave the Farmers State Bank corner at 11 A.M. This to take care of children and white personnel wishing to go to Sunday School." (NOTE: The ten o'clock bus formerly served the colored personnel.)[46]

Following the Klan march, a Mr. Jackson, who was being treated at the hospital for tuberculosis, wrote a letter to General Hines, protesting the march as well as the treatment of the approximately ninety hospital patients, and requesting protection for the black nurse-maids. When Colonel Stanley learned of his complaint, Mr. Jackson was discharged from the Tuskegee hospital and given transportation to Arizona before he had the opportunity to talk to representatives of the Department of Justice. Three of the black nurse-maids, Evelyn G. Robinson, Adella Woode, and Zelda H. Peck, were fired from the hospital for refusing to submit to the indignities placed upon them. The order, signed by Colonel Stanley, gave them less than twenty hours to leave the hospital property.[47]

On July 5 the national office of the NAACP wired President Harding, who was en route to Alaska, advising him of the critical situation at Tuskegee.

> National Association for the Advancement of Colored People representing one hundred thousand American citizens asks that Federal Troops be sent to Tuskegee, Alabama, to protect colored doctors sent to United States Veterans Hospital to care for Negro World War Veterans. Lives of these United States doctors and security of Tuskegee Institute have been threatened by masked mobs. Tuskegee Institute as internationally know agency making for inter-racial goodwill should have protection against lawless defiance of Government. We urge especially Federal protection for H. R. Moton successor to Booker T. Washington whose life has been threatened.[48]

Several days later, the NAACP sent a letter to J. Edgar Hoover at the Federal Bureau of Investigation informing him of the Klan march

1. Threats, Fear and Triumph

as well as the restrictions being placed on the hospital's black nursing staff. Part of that letter included:

> We have just received confidential information from Tuskegee that one Colonel Stanley, the present white head of the hospital, has notified the colored nurses at the government hospital that he does not wish them to have any contact whatever with the colored people of Tuskegee Institute. These nurses have absolutely no recreation or social outlet as the result of this announcement, and their positions as government employees are becoming increasingly difficult each day.
>
> After the Ku Klux Klan parade, noted in the newspapers, we are informed that several cars of hooded figures went to the hospital; that apparently instructions had been given to the guards to let them pass, as the hooded figures were saluted by the guards; the ropes taken down, and the Klansmen were permitted to enter upon the government reservations, and go through several of the buildings in search of John C. Calhoun, the colored man who was appointed as disbursing officers of the hospital.[49]

Although federal troops were not sent to Tuskegee, the Department of Justice's Bureau of Investigation was required to investigate the situation since Government property was threatened. Interviews were conducted with NAACP officials, Dr. M. O. Dumas of the National Medical Association, and two of the discharged nurse-maids.

John Calhoun had kept the unopened letter that had been delivered to him by Stanley in his pocket until two days later when he met in Atlanta with General Hines in who was on his way to Tuskegee to confer with the town's white citizens. The letter read: "WE UNDERSTAND YOU ARE REPORTING TO HOSPITAL TO ACCEPT DISBURSING OFFICERS' JOB. IF YOU VALUE YOUR WELFARE DO NOT TAKE THIS JOB BUT LEAVE AT ONCE FOR PARTS FROM WHENCE YOU CAME OR SUFFER THE CONSEQUENCES *** 'k' 'k' 'k.'"[50]

When Hines learned that Colonel Stanley had delivered this threat, he issued a formal reprimand and ordered Calhoun to return to the hospital to begin work. On July 24, after an official request was made by the NAACP for the immediate removal of Colonel Stanley, Hines was given presidential approval to make the change, replacing him with Dr. Charles M. Griffiths, a staff physician at the Veterans Bureau Hospital in Alexandria, Louisiana. Recognizing the need to have the cooperation of the town's white citizens, Hines agreed to work with a committee of local whites to reach a compromise. Despite the

The Tuskegee Veterans Hospital and Its Black Physicians

urging of the NAACP, who thought Hines had been intimidated and who pressured President Harding to follow through on his promise of a "complete colored staff," Dr. Moton acknowledged the need for a compromise. This change in Moton's position was influenced by a threat by W. W. Campbell, a trustee of Tuskegee Institute and a member of the white citizens' committee that had made another threat two months earlier. Campbell stated: "No steps [will] be taken that would disturb [the] institute if you would wire Hines that it is your desire [that] he cooperate in [the] fullest possible way with [the] white citizens of Tuskegee."[51]

While there was agreement between Hines and Moton that whites should remain in supervisory positions at the hospital for the present, Moton continued to press for the gradual replacement of white professional staff with blacks as vacancies occurred. Despite Moton's attempts at changing the racist attitudes of the white citizens of Tuskegee, which included arranging a meeting between the leaders of the National Medical Association and prominent white representatives, many blacks believed that he had endorsed the Jim Crow system of white supremacy and black subordination. W. E. B. DuBois wrote, "There is not reason in the world why white persons should not be appointed to the Tuskegee Hospital but the head of the hospital and the chief men in charge should, by every dictate of justice, be black men."[52]

Melvin Chisum wrote to General Frank T. Hines: "Those of us who have stood four square for a Negro personnel at the Tuskegee hospital represent the warp and woof of the true sentiment of the Race, and if, as I understand from your remarks yesterday, there be any black men of either high or low estate who are compromising in this situation and advising a part white staff at this hospital, then those persons do not represent the wishes and better judgment of their race."[53]

Moton's retreat to Washington, D.C., and his plan to work quietly behind the scenes further alienated many blacks, who accused him of running away from the conflict and not acting in the best interest of black citizens and veterans. There were signs that the NAACP was becoming disillusioned with Moton as early as May 1923, when one of its leaders, Shelby Davidson, complained that Moton was leading them to believe that he was pushing for a black staff, while at the same time

1. Threats, Fear and Triumph

siding with the white Southerners. Following several months of reports of double dealing by Moton, the organization withdrew their support of Moton and ceased further activity in the situation, but continued to be a visible advocate for black control of the hospital: "Major Moton ... said to the President and to General Hines ... that the heads of Tuskegee Institute were satisfied with a mixed staff and were willing for the hospital to be directed by white men just so long as there were colored doctors and nurses on the staff; that the officials at Washington should disregard the agitation of northern radicals who were merely trying to make propaganda out of the situation at Tuskegee."[54]

Throughout the spring and summer of 1923, African Americans protested that the Tuskegee Veterans Hospital be controlled and operated by blacks, arguing that if the facility and care were equal to those provided to whites, that black veterans would receive better treatment from members of their own race. Although Moton had retreated from a visible role in the battle, he enlisted the help of others to continue the pressure on the United States government. "It was necessary for Dr. Moton's friends to take up the fight through the press, and by telegrams to important Government officials with Dr. Moton left out, so that he can truthfully say that the colored people themselves, are making the fight for the hospital, and that because of the attitude of the people here, he is leaving the matter alone."[55]

Meanwhile, there was an increasing division among white Southerners over the integration of hospital personnel as evidenced by newspaper editorials that criticized the whites of Tuskegee. The *Mobile Register* commented that "the Ku Klux Klan demonstration in Tuskegee will probably make it harder for the government to recede from its purpose to place a wholly Negro staff in charge of the new hospital for Negro soldiers. While intended to show the strength of the opposition to the government's plan, it has also the aspects of a threat."[56] An editorial in the *Jackson Daily News* stated: "All this fuss and feathers at Tuskegee over the placing of Negro officers in a government hospital for the rehabilitation of Negro ex-servicemen strikes us as being downright silly. If the Negro soldiers are satisfied with Negro physicians, the white folks ought to have nothing to say about it."[57] The *Norfolk Virginia-Pilot* observed, "If there is a sound objection to staffing with competent colored personnel a hospital set aside exclusively for Negro patients ... nobody outside of Ku Klux Klan circles in Alabama seems to be aware of it."[58]

The Commission on Interracial Cooperation, an organization established in 1919 to promote race relations, also played a significant role in promoting black control of the hospital.[59] The white head of the commission, Will W. Alexander, convinced the social service commission of the Methodist Episcopal Church to issue a resolution condemning the Klan march and extending support for Tuskegee Institute. Alabama Power and Light were also persuaded by Alexander to denounce the Klan after several of its black employees refused to return to work on a company dam project because they feared for their safety.

Encouraged by the growing support of Southern newspapers as well as the support of Alabama's senior United States senator, Oscar W. Underwood, Hines ignored the protests of Tuskegee's white citizens and made the decision to proceed with a plan to give blacks all but the three top management positions at the hospital. He notified Stanley that the white officers currently holding positions would be given an opportunity to transfer to other stations as positions became available and those vacancies, with the exception of commanding officer, executive officer, and clinical director, would be filled by black people. This set off a protest by many blacks who saw it as "white management with colored subordinates."[60] Although the National Medical Association had been working to recruit black medical personnel, a resolution was passed by delegates at their annual conference, calling on black physicians to refuse positions at the Tuskegee Veterans Hospital "unless assured they are to serve under Negro officials."[61]

By mid–August, the nurses, attendants and laborers, constituting sixty percent of the staff, were black, and on August 15 it was announced that five black physicians had been assigned to Tuskegee. In June, the NMA had contacted Dr. Solomon Carter Fuller, a neuropathologist and America's first black psychiatrist, who was on the faculty of Boston University's School of Medicine. He was offered him a staff position at the Tuskegee VA hospital, with the opportunity to develop a neuropsychiatric unit. Declining the offer, which was repeated on two other occasions, Fuller agreed to recruit a group of black medical school graduates and supervise their training in neurology

1. Threats, Fear and Triumph

and psychiatry to prepare them for positions at Tuskegee.[62] Fuller later explained:

> About this time the Veterans' Hospital in Tuskegee was to be opened. I had been in correspondence with General Hines of the Veterans' Administration with respect to my taking over the organization of the Mental Department of the Institution, which, at the time I did not feel I could undertake for various reasons. There were two requests from the Veterans' Administration and the third which asked that, since I could not myself undertake the work, to select some promising young men and provide some clinical training in Psychiatry. This I was glad to do. I believed then and it has so proven this would be valuable experience.[63]

On November 21, 1923, when Fuller's students finally arrived at the Tuskegee hospital, progress toward the push for a black-operated facility had been made. Of the hospital's 247 employees caring for 226 patients, eighteen were African American. Racial tensions in the town over the hospital had lessoned, with the attention of its residents focused on the new railroad and its potential effect on the area's economy. Both Major Moton and Dr. Kenney had returned, the physician reporting that "it appears that the unpleasant and trying experience which we have sustained here with reference to the Veterans' Hospital will, 'ere long, be past history."[64]

2

Health Care for Black Veterans

Medical Care

Prior to World War I, the federal government provided no system of medical care to veterans. Pensions for disabled veterans had been provided since 1636, when the English colonies in North America passed a law that paid money to those who were disabled in the colonies' defense against Native Americans. Soon after the ratification of the U.S. Constitution in 1789, the first federal pension legislation was passed and by 1808, all veterans programs were administered by the Bureau of Pensions under the secretary of war. The programs were later placed under the secretary of the navy in the Office of Pensions, which was renamed the Bureau of Pensions, and assigned to the new Department of the Interior in 1850. With the passage of the General Pension Act of 1862, disability payments became available for veterans as well as for widows, children and dependent relatives. The law covered military service in time of peace as well as during war and for the first time, included compensation for diseases such as tuberculosis incurred while in the service.[1]

In the early 1800s, under the Marine Hospital Service Act of 1798, the United States government began to open marine hospitals on the Atlantic coast and on inland waterways for the medical care of merchant seaman. Administered by what came to be called the U.S. Public Health Service, Marine hospitals, soldiers' homes, the U.S. Naval Home in Philadelphia, St. Elizabeth's Hospital in Washington, D.C., and some active-duty army and navy hospitals provided medical care

2. Health Care for Black Veterans

for veterans on an as-needed basis. The National Asylum for Disabled Volunteer Soldiers was authorized by Congress in 1865 to establish residences that provided room and board and some medical care to disabled and indigent veterans. Renamed the National Home for Disabled Volunteer Soldiers in 1873, the program cared for veterans of the Mexican, Civil, Indian and Spanish-American wars as well as for noncombat veterans.[2]

During the Civil War, blacks suffered proportionately heavier casualties than whites because medical care was both primitive and scarce for them. One United States Colored Troops (USCT) doctor stated, "Very few surgeons will do precisely the same for blacks as they would for whites."[3] It was difficult to find qualified white surgeons to serve with black troops and the War Department was reluctant to commission available black physicians. Only eight black physicians were appointed surgeons to the army.[4] Seven of those served in Washington, D.C., hospitals. One, Alexander T. Augusta, was the first African American to hold a medical commission in the U.S. army and to be promoted to lieutenant colonel, U.S.V., for faithful and meritorious service. He was also the first African American officer to be buried in Arlington National Cemetery. As the senior surgeon with the 7th U.S. Colored Infantry stationed at Camp Stanton, Maryland, Dr. Augusta outranked the white surgeons. Two of the white assistant surgeons of the 9th and 19th regiments of black infantry expressed their resentment at having to take commands from a black man, and wrote to President Lincoln:

> When we made application for position on the Colored Service, the understanding was universal that all commissioned officers were to be white men. Judge of our surprise when, upon joining our respective regiments, we found that the Senior Surgeon of the Command was a Negro.
> We claim to be behind no one, in a desire for the elevation and improvement of the colored race in this Country, and we are willing to sacrifice much in so grand a cause, as our present positions may testify. But we cannot in any cause, willingly compromise what we consider a proper self-respect; nor do we deem that the interests of either the country or of the colored race, can demand this of us. Such degradation, we believe to be involved in our voluntarily continuing in the service, as subordinate to a colored officer. We therefore most respectively, yet earnestly request that this unexpected, unusual, and most unpleasant relationship in which we have been placed, may in some way be terminated.[5]

The Tuskegee Veterans Hospital and Its Black Physicians

As a result of the complaints by the white surgeons, Dr. Augusta was placed on detached service, examining black recruits. At the end of the war, seven other black physicians, John Van Surly deGrass, Charles Purvis, Alpheus Tucker, John Rapier, William Ellis, Anderson Abbott, and William Powell, Jr., remained on active duty providing care for the 180,000 black American servicemen who served in the conflict.[6]

When America entered into World War I, it was the first time that a large number of combat victims survived and it was decided to extend medical treatment of the returning troops. As a result, Congress enacted legislation in 1917 amending the War Risk Law that made injured military personnel eligible to receive medical, surgical, and hospital services at facilities operated by the United States government. The amended law also offered government-subsidized life insurance for veterans and paved the way for rehabilitation and vocational training for veterans with dismemberment, sight, hearing, and other permanent disabilities.[7] To establish a national system of health care for veterans, the Veterans Bureau was created in 1921. Although the Public Health Service operated a few hospitals, most medical care for veterans was being provided in armed services hospitals. The 204,000 wounded World War I veterans proved to be too much of a burden for the military hospitals, resulting in the authorization of new hospitals and the use of private hospitals by contract. The bureau, later renamed the Veterans Administration, consolidated veterans affairs and the following year took control of public service hospitals that provided care to veterans.

As in previous wars, the War Department was reluctant to commission black physicians during World War I, and black health professionals had to overcome many obstacles in order to serve their country. As a result of an urgent appeal for physicians to enlist in the Medical Reserve Corps by the War Department in the summer of 1917, white physicians who responded were at once commissioned and assigned to active duty. At the same time, 200 of the estimated 300 black physicians who had been commissioned had not been assigned to active duty nor was there any evidence that the Department of the Surgeon General had plans to use them.[8]

In an attempt to do his part for the war effort, Dr. Solomon Carter Fuller, the African American neuropsychiatrist who would later prepare

2. Health Care for Black Veterans

black physicians to work at the Tuskegee Veterans Hospital, offered his services. A letter from the War Department dated August 1, 1918, written in response to his offer to serve made the case that his race would be an obstacle in attaining military rank.

> My dear Dr. Fuller:
>
> The need for your services continues. On the other hand, there are some obstacles in the way of obtaining your services. I find that it would not be possible to grant you a commission until you have been naturalized.
>
> Under a law recently passed, one who is not now a citizen can be immediately naturalized upon enlisting in the Army. We are utilizing this law in obtaining commissions for a number of men. The process is for the man to enlist in the Army as a private. We usually have him do this here in Washington, in order that, as soon as he is enlisted, we can order him to St. Elizabeth's Hospital, where the situation is understood. The man is then given a ten day leave of absence. During these ten days his naturalization is completed and his application for a commission put through. By the time it is necessary for him to report back to duty, he usually has his commission, and goes out as an officer. We have recently succeeded in doing this in two cases.
>
> The other obstacle is unfortunately in regard to race. I am sure you wish one to speak frankly on this matter, as you know my own personal feelings. It is not likely that a commission higher than that of lieutenant could be granted to you on the start. It is possible that you might obtain a captaincy, but this is doubtful. It is not likely that it would ever be possible for you to obtain a commission higher than that of captain.
>
> This might handicap you somewhat in your work in the Army, but I think not seriously. If, under these conditions, you feel that you can apply, you may be sure that you will be most cordially welcomed by this division. Your services are needed, and you would receive every support from us.
>
> Sincerely,
> Frankwood E. Williams, Major, M.R.C.
> Office of the Surgeon General
> War Department
> Washington, D.C.

Fuller's reply, dated August 5, 1918, was as follows:

> My dear Dr. Williams:
>
> The very frank tone of your letter of August 1, is greatly appreciated. The method for overcoming the first obstacle which you mentioned, namely by enlisting as a private and under the new law attaining citizenship within a short period is satisfactory. This I would gladly undertake.
>
> The other obstacle, however, is something more than an obstacle, as ordinarily

The Tuskegee Veterans Hospital and Its Black Physicians

understood; apparently it is an impasse infranchissable (sic). The conditions laid down with this latter obstacle seem to preclude the possibility of rendering the sort of service for which by training experience, I am best qualified. Needless to add my regrets, but in the face of the clearly defined limitations imposed for me, I believe the work could be more effectively performed by one with fewer handicaps.

You will understand, I am sure, that to serve effectively the group of men in the army with whom I would be identified, would be the greatest possible satisfaction, but if I cannot serve them effectively—and I do not see how this can be done under "conditions"—the only course open to me with respect to your offer must be obvious. I feel, therefore, that in my present position as pathologist and director of clinical psychiatry, in an established institution administering to the public need, the opportunity for service of a worth while character is greater than in the very restricted field which your letter outlines.

Believe me.

Very sincerely yours,
Dr. Solomon Carter Fuller[9]

An investigation into this state of affairs found that the Department of the Surgeon General had adopted a policy not to issue any new commissions to black physicians, nor to assign to active duty to those who had already been commissioned, but were not yet assigned.[10] Following an intense debate at their national convention in Richmond, Virginia, the NMA passed a set of declarations on August 29, 1918, that objected to the policy which barred many black physicians from providing medical services to the military and requested that they be given consideration for service in the Medical Reserve Corps based on their merit as physicians. Initial efforts by the NMA to arrange a meeting with government officials and legislators in order to discuss the issues addressed in the declarations were unsuccessful, as seen in the following letter dated November 14, 1918.

Dr. G. E. Cannon
Chairman, Executive Board
National Medical Association
Jersey City, New Jersey

My dear Dr. Cannon:

In reply to your letter of November 9, addressed to General Ireland, I am directed to say that this Department has not been in any way prejudiced against the appointment of colored medical officers. As many such officers have been assigned as circumstances would permit.

2. Health Care for Black Veterans

Since the Student's Army Training Corps was formed, the Department has taken advantage of the opportunity to assign as many additional colored medical officers as the facts warranted. It is quite impracticable to assign colored officers to organizations where all of the other officers are white.

To do so would be embarrassing to all concerned.

General Ireland has given this matter his close personal attention since he assumed the office of Surgeon General.

Yours very truly,
R. B. Miller
Colonel, Medical Corps, U. S. A.
Office of the Surgeon General[11]

During the next few months, the NMA distributed 1500 copies of the declarations throughout the country, making sure that copies were sent to congressmen, governors and other government officials. Finally, on December 12, the Executive Committee of the NMA met with the third assistant secretary of war, Frederick Keppel, to register their protest against the discrimination practiced against black physicians and to ask that they, as well as black dentists and nurses, be given equal consideration in the U.S. army.

As a result of the NMA's efforts, a large number of black physicians eventually served as medical officers with the black combatant organizations in France. In the 92nd Division, black medical officers were on duty with the 365th, 366th, 367th and 368th Infantry Regiments; the 349th, 350th and 351st Machine Gun Battalions; the 317th Regiment of Engineers; the 325th Field Signal Battalion; the 365th, 366th, 367th and 368th Field Hospital; and ambulance companies and the division supply train and military police. Although the division surgeon, division sanitary inspector, regimental surgeons and the commanding officers of the field hospitals were white, the majority of the remaining medical officers were black, including the commanding officers of all of the ambulance companies and the surgeons of many of the battalions. In the 93rd Division, the regiment surgeon of the 370th Infantry and medical officers who served with the 369th and 372nd Infantry regiments were black.[12]

Prior to the opening of the Tuskegee Veterans Hospital, disabled black veterans received inferior health care, especially in the South. Although they had fought America's wars alongside white soldiers, many African Americans were refused admission to veterans hospitals

The Tuskegee Veterans Hospital and Its Black Physicians

and those veterans who were fortunate to receive any care at all found segregation and unequal treatment in wards of hospitals that were located at great distances from their homes and not suitable for the prolonged periods of rehabilitation for battle casualties.

Following the abolition of slavery in 1865, the federal government established the Freedman's Bureau to assume responsibility for the medical care of former slaves who had previously received care from plantation owners. Although the Freedman's Bureau hospitals, set up in the South and in neighboring states, provided some medical care to freed slaves who migrated from the plantations to urban areas, the organization's lack of funding and poor management made it difficult to meet the medical needs of five million former slaves.[13]

By 1872, only one of the Freedman's Bureau's forty-five hospitals remained open. A special Congressional mandate allowed the Washington, D.C., facility to operate as Freedman's Hospital under the direction of the War Department. As a military hospital, the facility provided care to all veterans, regardless of color. Dr. Augusta was placed in charge during the first year, becoming the first African American physician to head a hospital in the United States. The hospital was later transferred from the War Department to the Department of the Interior and became an asylum for ailing refugees of the emancipation. In 1969, the Freedmen's Hospital became a part of Howard University and was renamed Howard University Hospital during the Civil Rights era in the 20th century.

In 1865, Congress established the National Home for Disabled Volunteer Soldiers to provide residential long term care for disabled veterans.[14,15] The home was initially open to any Union soldier with a service-connected injury, offering recreational opportunities and jobs. Confederate veterans were excluded from admission at National Home branches, but were accepted at similar homes that were funded and managed by several states. By 1884, membership had been expanded to include any honorably discharged veteran who could not support himself due to a service-related disability. Black veterans were initially allowed membership at the National Home branches, which established a policy of racial equality. But the level of equality decreased following the Civil War, and while African Americans continued to be allowed admission, living quarters were segregated, with separate barracks and dining facilities. Although ten percent of the Union army was African American, by 1900 only two and one-half percent of the residents at the National Home branches were black. The homes were closed in the 1950s when the last Civil War veteran died.

Treatment of Mental Disorders

Before the Civil War, blacks who were thought to be mentally ill were excluded from asylums or segregated within an institution and often placed in almshouses and jails. Worcester Hospital in Massachusetts, Virginia's Eastern Lunatic Asylum, and the South Carolina Lunatic Asylum were among those insane asylums providing separate wings for black patients.[16] The care provided in these asylums applied only to free Negroes, with the exception of the South Carolina facility that operated under an ordinance passed in 1848 by the legislature entitled "An Act to Authorize the Admission of Persons of Color into the Lunatic Asylum." Mentally ill slaves were supposed to be taken care of by their owners on their plantations.

The roles that both biology and culture played in the etiology of mental illness among African Americans were given credit for the increase in reports of insanity among blacks. Many colonial psychiatrists believed that an inferior physiology was the determinative factor in the etiology of mental illness among African Americans. This theory was given credibility by the work of J. C. Carothers, an American psychiatrist living in Kenya, who maintained that the brains of Africans were underdeveloped compared with those of Europeans.[17]

Pre–Civil War American psychiatrists argued that insanity accompanied civilization and that this condition existed only in advanced, sophisticated societies. Since African and American Indian societies were considered savage cultures without intellectual or material attainment, African Americans, being only a few generations removed from their African roots, were thought to be immune from serious mental disorders. It was also assumed by psychiatrists that while few slaves experienced mental illnesses, free blacks would exhibit more signs of mental disorder as a result of their experiences with civilization. This belief was reinforced with the publication of the *United States Census*

The Tuskegee Veterans Hospital and Its Black Physicians

Report of 1840, which included statistical tables illustrating the distribution of the insane by race and state. The document reported that the incidence of insanity among free blacks was eleven times greater than among slaves, with higher rates in the Northern states which had larger populations of free blacks.[18] Although the census was found to contain gross errors and contradictions by Dr. Edward Jarvis, a Massachusetts physician and one of the country's leading statisticians, the statistics were used by proslavery propagandists to argue that slavery protected the mental health of blacks by sheltering them from the anxieties, intemperance, and other excesses of civilization. Secretary of State John C. Calhoun, when requested by Congress to reexamine the census, brought back the Southern census-taker who had been in charge of the original enumeration as an expert witness who successfully defended the figures and refused to admit error.

The belief that emancipation was traumatic for enslaved blacks became a convincing assumption as medical and mental health professionals struggled with what they perceived to be an increase in cases of insanity among African Americans in the late nineteenth century. Citing the rise in the incidence of diseases such as tuberculosis and syphilis as evidence that freedom had a deleterious effect upon blacks, they attributed the increase in physical and mental illness to their removal from the paternalistic relationship of slavery and their exposure to the stress and demands of modern civilization.

The Anglo-American psychiatric community also believed that mentally ill whites and blacks manifested different pathologies. Observations of disproportionate cases of mania among black asylum inmates fueled the preconceptions that black "madness" was of a more violent nature than that of whites with a mental illness. This difference was characterized by black insanity's "debasing nature" and an "increase of the animal propensities" and was evidenced by the predisposition of blacks toward mania and the greater prevalence of melancholia among whites.

> The insane negro is combative and homicidal, but suicidal tendencies rarely exist. Dementia and melancholia are common, but the most frequent forms met with can best be characterized as moral or emotional, fraught with hallucinations and delusions. The superstition and credulity of the negro render his untutored mind ripe for ideas and impressions calculated to dethrone his reason,

2. Health Care for Black Veterans

and he falls an easy victim to fear, fright, rage, jealousy, ambition, religious fanaticism, political commotions, and all phases of undue excitement coincident with his surroundings.[19]

The popular belief in black hypersexuality was also linked to a supposed propensity to mania. Physicians perpetuated the myth that blacks were more sexually active than whites and attributed the incidence of syphilis among this population to sexual promiscuity and physical inferiority.[20]

By the early 1900s, due to the clinical work of Emil Kraepelin, which led to the classification of mental illnesses, mania and melancholia were understood to be mental states that were often part of a cycle of a manic-depressive disorder. This conception resulted in a dispute over the extent to which African Americans suffered from this newly identified psychosis. In a study of 800 black and white women admitted to St. Elizabeth's Hospital in Washington, D.C., from 1909 to 1914, a diagnosis of manic-depressive disorder was rare among the black patients.[21] Conflicting results were found in another study which examined the records of almost 3000 black men and women admitted to the Georgia State Sanitarium between 1910 and 1915 and found a higher incidence of manic-depressive disorder among blacks than whites.[22]

St. Elizabeth's opened as the Government Hospital for the Insane in 1855 in Washington, D.C., to house and treat individuals who were judged mentally ill while under federal jurisdiction.[23] The asylum's admissions included active-duty members and veterans of the army, navy, and merchant marines, in addition to American citizens living in or traveling through U.S. territories, American Indians residing on reservations, and inmates of federal and state penitentiaries. The African American inmate population included soldiers, sailors and veterans as well as residents of the District of Columbia, and were housed in a separate lodge. The prevailing treatment theory of the nineteenth century dictated that the insane be grouped according to their pathology, symptoms and behavior, in addition to race, ethnicity, gender and class. While the hospital's first superintendent, Charles H. Nichols, believed that it was the government's responsibility to treat mentally ill blacks, he realized that housing black and white patients in close proximity to one another would promote hostility and hinder

The Tuskegee Veterans Hospital and Its Black Physicians

treatment.[24] The lodge was positioned several hundred feet from the main building and initially housed both men and women. Within four years, the increase in the number of black patients led to funding by Congress that resulted in the building of a separate lodge for black men located between the main building and the stables. St. Elizabeth's practice of segregation was maintained until the 1950s.

With the emancipation of the slaves following the Civil War, states were faced with the responsibility for providing residential care for mentally ill blacks and began to admit them to asylums. Segregation remained the norm, with Northern and Western states placing black patients in separate rooms or small wards and Southern states designating special wings or buildings for blacks. In 1869, the first institution to be devoted exclusively to the care of blacks declared to be mentally insane was established near Richmond, Virginia. The hospital, Howard's Grove Asylum, later renamed the Central State Hospital, was relocated in Petersburg and opened in 1885.[25] By 1912, four states—Alabama, Maryland, North Carolina, and Virginia—had mental hospitals specifically designated for blacks.

There is little mention of military psychiatry in the literature of military medicine prior to World War I. Only a few pages on mental and nervous diseases are included in the official medical and surgical history of the Civil War and the subject is completely omitted in the volume *Military, Medical and Surgical Essays*, prepared for the U.S. Sanitary Commission, edited by Surgeon General William A. Hammond and published in 1864.[26] The subject of military psychiatry rarely appeared in the leading psychiatric journal, the *American Journal of Insanity*, or in presentations read at the annual meeting of the Association of Medical Superintendents of American Institutions for the Insane during the war years. It was the neurologists, not the psychiatrists, who participated in military medicine and most of the psychiatric literature pertaining to the Civil War appeared in journals of general medicine.

The psychiatric experiences of World War I gave mental health professionals an opportunity to observe the effects of a war which surpassed all others both in its vast proportions and in its unprecedented mass destruction. The tensions of World War I brought to the surface many of the problems of mental illness that had been hidden

2. Health Care for Black Veterans

or underestimated in peacetime, intensifying the need for a large scale mental health program in the military.

One of the first acts of the Federal Government following United States' entry into the war was the creation of a division of neurology and psychiatry within the surgeon general's office.[27] The division's functions were (1) to prepare for the examination of recruits in the mobilization camps in order to screen for those who may not be suitable for military duty due to neuropathic or psychiatric conditions; (2) to prepare adequate facilities for the observation, treatment and care of soldiers with nervous or mental diseases pending discharge; (3) to prepare for the treatment of soldiers in the American Expeditionary Forces (AEF) who become incapacitated because of nervous or mental disease; and (4) to prepare for the continued treatment and final disposition of soldiers sent home.

The task of organizing a psychiatric branch in the Army Medical Corps was assigned to the National Committee for Mental Hygiene. The committee's medical director, Dr. Thomas W. Salmon, became chief of psychiatry in the AEF and helped to develop a system of hospital treatment for members of the forces who required psychiatric care. He also began psychiatric screening of draft registrants and set up a program to rehabilitate returning soldiers with mental disorders. Neither the military nor the American health care system had the treatment programs necessary to provide care for the estimated 70,000 World War I veterans diagnosed with neuropsychiatric disabilities.[28] To meet the needs of this population, neuropsychiatric wards were established in general hospitals throughout the country, with the more serious psychotic soldiers admitted to St. Elizabeth's Hospital in Washington, D.C. The majority of those who were disabled as a result of a neuropsychiatric disorder, became wards of the United States Public Health Service, and eventually were cared for by the Veterans Bureau.

The modern artillery firepower used in World War I resulted in the identification of a new type of battle injury that left no visible wounds. The diagnosis of "shell shock" first appeared in the British medical journal *The Lancet* in 1916, six months after the beginning of the war.[29] In the article, it was reported that three soldiers who had each been exposed to exploding shells, exhibited symptoms of "reduced visual fields," loss of smell and taste, and some memory loss. Originally

The Tuskegee Veterans Hospital and Its Black Physicians

thought to be related to the severe concussive motion of the shaken soldier's brain, it was later believed that a majority of shell shock cases were the emotional reactions to the horrors of trench warfare, reflecting the recent advances in psychiatry. Also known as neurasthenia and war neurosis, the condition presented with an assortment of symptoms ranging from anxiety, exaggerated startled response and tremors to the more debilitating nightmares, hallucinations, delusions, withdrawal, and catatonia. By 1917, medical officers were directed to avoid the term "shell shock," using instead the diagnosis "Not Yet Diagnosed (Nervous)." The soldier was then transferred to a psychiatric unit and assessed by a clinical specialist. If the soldier was found to be suffering from either "shell shock (wound)" or "shell shock (sick)," he was transferred to a treatment center in Britain or France for recovery and then either discharged or returned to the front. The pressure to deny or minimize the severity of the neuroses affecting an increasing number of soldiers was re-enforced by recommendations for treatment that were made in a report by the chief of the Division of Neurology and Psychiatry in the surgeon general's office, who served as the consultant in neuropsychiatry for the AEF.

Check the development of neurosis by denying its existence at the start.

> Each army should have its own center of a capacity of at least one and a half beds to each 1,000 troops. It should keep its patients two or three weeks if necessary, and should be entirely independent of any hospital or the communication or base.
>
> The treatment of the patients should be calmative and restorative and any appearance of such symptoms as tremors, paralysis, etc. should be rigidly discouraged. This idea should run through the whole personnel of the hospital.
>
> At first it should be effected by gentle persuasion but, if the patients persist in the production of hysterical symptoms, sterner measures should be resorted to.
>
> It is not considered desirable to send patients of this class to convalescent camps.
>
> It would be better for them to have leaves, and the threat to cut off the leave might persuade many to suppress the self-indulgence which is so often the neurosis and give up their symptoms. Isolation and strong faradization might also be employed with advantage at this stage.[30]

The psychoneuroses constituted the most significant challenge in World War I psychiatry. In the United States, the more common

2. Health Care for Black Veterans

psychoneuroses among white soldiers were neurasthenia, a pattern of symptoms often linked to depression, and psychasthenia, characterized by phobias, obsessions and compulsions, or excessive anxieties. These diagnoses are no longer used in psychiatry. In black soldiers, hysteria and stammering were cited as primary symptoms in over 70 percent of the neurotic reactions.

Beginning with World War I, many black veterans were labeled by the Veterans Administration as "behavioral disorders" or "bad conduct cases," conditions thought to have resulted from syphilis of the central nervous system.[31] This misdiagnosis rendered black veterans ineligible for benefits and allowed for whites to be appointed as their guardians with fiscal responsibility.

St. Elizabeth's Hospital became the primary destination for psychotic soldiers. As the numbers increased, the capacity of the government hospital was unable to meet the demand. As a result, some of the patients were sent to the neuropsychiatric wards of base hospitals, while less serious cases were returned to their communities. Many, through the cooperation between the National Committee for Mental Hygiene and several state hospitals, were cared for in state mental hospitals. The majority of the disabled soldiers suffering from neuropsychiatric illnesses became wards of the United States Public Health Service and were eventually cared for by the Veterans Bureau.[32]

3

Responding to the Call for Black Physicians at the Tuskegee Veterans Hospital

Opportunities for Black Physicians

In 1900, there were seven black medical schools in addition to several proprietary schools in Washington, D.C., that offered evening programs primarily for federal employees who had full-time jobs.[1] By 1920 there were 3,885 black physicians in the United States, but the number of black medical schools had decreased as a result of the implementation of recommendations made by the Flexner Report. The report, issued in 1910 by the Carnegie Foundation for the Advancement of Teaching, raised standards for medical education which led to the closing of all but two black medical schools, leaving only Howard and Meharry.[2] Like most professions, medical training was segregated and the majority of black physicians attended black medical schools. According to Abraham Flexner in *Medical Education in the United States and Canada*,

> The practice of the Negro doctor will be limited to his own race, which in turn will be cared for better by good Negro physicians than by poor white ones. But the physical well-being of the Negro is not only of moment to the Negro himself. Ten million of them live in close contact with sixty million whites. Not only does the Negro himself suffer from hookworm and tuberculosis; he communicates them to his white neighbors, precisely as the ignorant and unfortunate white contaminates him. Self-protection not less than humanity offers

3. Black Physicians at the Tuskegee Hospital

weighty counsel in this matter; self-interest seconds philanthropy. The Negro must be educated not only for his sake, but for ours. He is, as far as human eye can see, a permanent factor in the nation. He has his rights and due and value as an individual; but he has, besides the tremendous importance that belongs to a potential source of infection and contagion.

The pioneer work in educating the race to know and practice fundamental hygienic principles must be done largely by the Negro doctor and the Negro nurse. It is important they both be sensibly and effectively trained at the level at which their services are now important. The Negro is perhaps more easily 'taken in' than the white; and as his means of extricating himself from a blunder are limited, it is all the more cruel to abuse his ignorance through any sort of pretense. A well-taught Negro sanitarian will be immensely useful; an essentially untrained Negro wearing an M. D. degree is dangerous.[3]

Flexner's model of institutional racism in health care limited the black physician's practice of medicine to the African American population, thus focusing their education on the principles of hygiene rather than the techniques of surgery and training in medical specialties. According to Flexner, their place in American medicine would be to serve as protectors of the white population by preventing the spread of TB and other infections seen as "black" health diseases.

Recommended by the American Medical Association's Council on Medical Education in 1905, clinical training in the form of internships and other forms of post graduate instruction became an integral component in the education of physicians.[4] These reforms created a new dilemma for black medical personnel. Opportunities for training were limited due to the racial discrimination practiced by most predominately white hospitals and the inability of the few small black hospitals with scarce resources to provide approved training programs. During the Reconstruction period, segregated hospitals were established, many of them sponsored by whites who were motivated for both humanitarian reasons and by the belief that African Americans were carriers of disease that posed a threat to white people. Most of these segregated hospitals were in the South, where restricted racial codes and traditions resulted in limited and lower quality care to its black population. In response to the racism in American medicine, black physicians, educational institutions, churches and fraternal organizations began to establish hospitals during the end of the nineteenth and the beginning of the twentieth centuries. These black-controlled health

The Tuskegee Veterans Hospital and Its Black Physicians

care facilities provided opportunities not often available to black physicians for training, staff privileges, and learning about the latest developments in medicine.[5]

An estimated 202 black hospitals existed in 1923, with only six offering internships and none with residency programs. Those black medical students who were accepted for clinical training at "integrated" facilities often found that they were excluded from administering care to white patients because of objections from patients and from some administrators.[6] Finding it especially difficult to receive clinical experience in obstetrics and gynecology, some found it necessary to enroll at black medical schools such as Howard or Meharry in order to complete their clinical training.

The black physician encountered the same obstacles in securing hospital staff appointments as he met in obtaining medical education. Hospitals that admitted black patients often did not grant staff privileges to black physicians. The inability to follow their patients in the hospital forced many African American physicians to turn over their black patients to white physicians. Finding hospital positions closed to

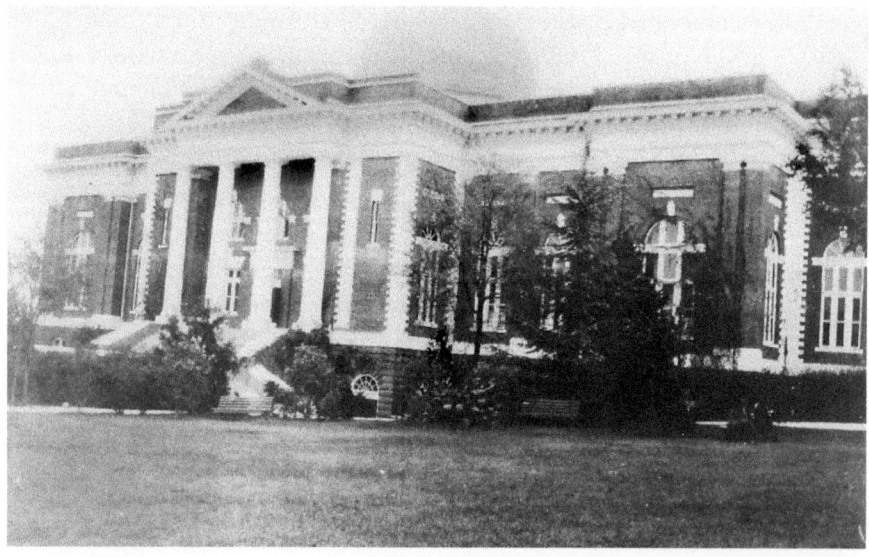

Tuskegee Veterans Hospital, 1923 (Tuskegee University Archives, Tuskegee, Alabama).

3. Black Physicians at the Tuskegee Hospital

them throughout the country, many developed a number of small proprietary, semi-proprietary, and later voluntary hospitals throughout the South and in major cities in the North. These were often the only places in which they could gain hospital experience and practice medicine.

In addition to a degree from an accredited medical school and successful completion of an approved residency program, membership in the local medical society was also required for staff privileges at most hospitals. As a step toward the improvement of professional status for black physicians, the National Medical Association was established in 1895, following their unsuccessful attempts to gain membership in the American Medical Association (AMA). Composed of liberal white physicians, mostly members of the Howard medical faculty and black physicians, the group attempted to have its delegates recognized at the twenty-first annual convention of the AMA, which was held that year in Washington, D.C. The AMA refused to recognize the delegates of the National Medical Association and passed a resolution that stated, "It has been distinctly stated and proved that the consideration of race and color has had nothing whatsoever to do with the decision of the question of the reception of the Washington delegates."[7] It was at this meeting that the AMA also affirmed the states rights policy, by refusing to take any steps to secure membership for black doctors in affiliated county and state medical societies in states where they were excluded. This policy remained in effect for eighty years until the organization's 1950 San Francisco convention, where the AMA requested member societies having racially restrictive membership provisions to review those provisions in light of current social views, with consideration for their removal.

The NMA held annual meetings that provided a forum for the presentation of scientific papers and clinical demonstrations as well as the latest developments in medical practice and education. In 1909, the NMA began publication of the *Journal of the National Medical Association*, which offered members the opportunity to publish their scientific and clinical research. As the organization's membership grew, local medical societies were established and by 1914, there were forty local societies throughout the country.

Concerned about the difficulties encountered by black physicians in obtaining access to quality hospitals as well as meeting the new standards set by the American Medical Association and the American College of Surgeons, the NMA established the National Hospital Association (NHA) in 1923. Operating under the direction of the NMA, the organization's role was to establish and monitor standards of education and quality in black hospitals. While condemning racial segregation in principle, the organizations were forced to shape their policies according to the reality of discrimination in the medical field, which necessitated the establishment of separate facilities for African Americans.

Solomon Carter Fuller's Challenge and Commitment

Although Solomon Carter Fuller declined the Veterans Administration's offer to join the staff at Tuskegee, he agreed to train a small group of recent African American medical school graduates in neuropsychiatry who were to become the nucleus of that service at the hospital. Acknowledged and respected for his research and teaching in the field of neuroscience and psychiatry, Fuller's memories and experiences of fighting racism in his efforts to obtain a medical degree and training were still fresh. Born in Liberia, the grandson of an American slave, John Lewis Fuller, who bought his freedom and left the United States for a better life in west Africa, Fuller came to the United States in 1889 with the dream of becoming a physician.[8] He planned to stay just until he became qualified to practice medicine and then to return to Liberia to continue his grandparents' medical missionary work. After graduating from Livingston College, a black college in Salisbury, North Carolina, affiliated with the African Methodist Episcopal Church, he was admitted to the Long Island College Hospital's medical degree program. In 1894, shortly after he began his studies, Fuller transferred to Boston University School of Medicine. Most American medical schools did not accept African American students at that time, but the American Colonization Society, with the goal of encouraging the migration of blacks to Liberia, would sponsor the

3. Black Physicians at the Tuskegee Hospital

medical training of a few with the understanding that they would go to Liberia to practice. It was reported that Fuller was offered financial assistance through this program, but refused to accept the funds under this condition.[9]

Fuller's experience in the pathology of syphilis as well as his interest in what was then known as shell shock, gave him the expertise to prepare the medical trainees to treat the veterans who would be admitted to the Tuskegee hospital. The reputation of Fuller's pathology laboratory at Westborough State Hospital was well known, and for many years it was one of only two laboratories in Massachusetts that did the analyses for the Wasserman tests for syphilis for the state hospitals. In an undated paper written by Fuller, entitled "Anatomical Findings of General Paresis and Multiple Sclerosis in the Same Case," he documented the results of an autopsy performed on a female patient, originally diagnosed with multiple sclerosis, where he found clinical signs of syphilis.

> Based upon the clinical and anatomical data furnished by this case, there has been some speculation in the mind of the writer as to whether the great malefactor syphilis may not under certain favorable conditions serve as a genetic factor for multiple sclerosis and in the discussion some consideration has been given those speculations…. It is well to keep in mind that both multiple sclerosis and paresis are common organic nervous afflictions, that both occur in comparatively young people and have their inception at an even earlier period of life. It is, therefore, conceivable that a young multiple sclerotic person, at a period before the disease had caused any serious disturbance, could acquire syphilis and later exhibit simultaneously the characteristic anatomical lesions.[10]

During World War I, Fuller had developed an interest in the study of the disturbance to the nervous system related to battle. Known as "shell shock," it was also referred to as "battle fatigue," "conversion hysteria," and "exhaustion neurosis" and was initially deemed to be a physical injury. But by 1916, military and medical experts were convinced that the characteristic symptoms—trembling, headache, ringing in the ear, dizziness, poor concentration, confusion, loss of memory and sleep disorders were psychological manifestations precipitated by the stress of war.[11] It was Fuller's opinion that it was the government's responsibility to rehabilitate veterans suffering from combat induced mental disorders.[12]

The Tuskegee Veterans Hospital and Its Black Physicians

In addition to his work as a neuropathologist, Fuller had become interested in those psychological disorders that appeared to have no organic cause. This led him to explore functional psychological conditions and the effects that the psychotherapy pioneered by Sigmund Freud and others in the mental health field might have on these disorders. As one of the first proponents of the new psychoanalytic theories, Fuller began practicing psychiatry in the early 1900s, integrating the new psychology in the treatment of such mental disorders as schizophrenia and manic depression.

Fuller transcended science into practice, establishing himself as America's first black psychiatrist in 1919. The war had ended and he had resigned from Westborough State Hospital, transferring his research activities to Boston. He continued his clinical instruction in the Department of Neurology and Psychiatry at Boston University's School of Medicine and his position as a consulting neurologist at Massachusetts Memorial Hospital. He also maintained a small psychiatry practice in his home in Framingham as well as in his Boston office, treating patients regardless of their color or ability to pay.

To staff the Tuskegee Veterans Hospital with qualified black physicians, the National Medical Association was requested to submit a list of candidates from its membership within sixty days. The identification and selection process proved difficult as there were few trained qualified black physicians. Fuller succeeded in recruiting and training four graduating medical students, three from Boston University and one from Harvard. With only a few weeks to provide training in neuropsychiatry, Fuller enlisted the help of two of his Boston colleagues, Dr. C. Macfie Campbell and Dr. John P. Sutherland.

Dr. Sutherland was a professor of anatomy at Boston University Medical School and had worked on several research projects with Fuller, including the investigation of the use of urine analysis to determine indicators of morphine and opium addiction.[13]

Dr. Campbell had recently become the director of the Massachusetts Psychiatric Institute, located within the Boston Psychopathic Hospital, following the death of Dr. Southard in 1920. Like Fuller, he had studied neurology and psychiatry in Germany, working in Franz Nissl's Heidelberg laboratory in 1903.

3. Black Physicians at the Tuskegee Hospital

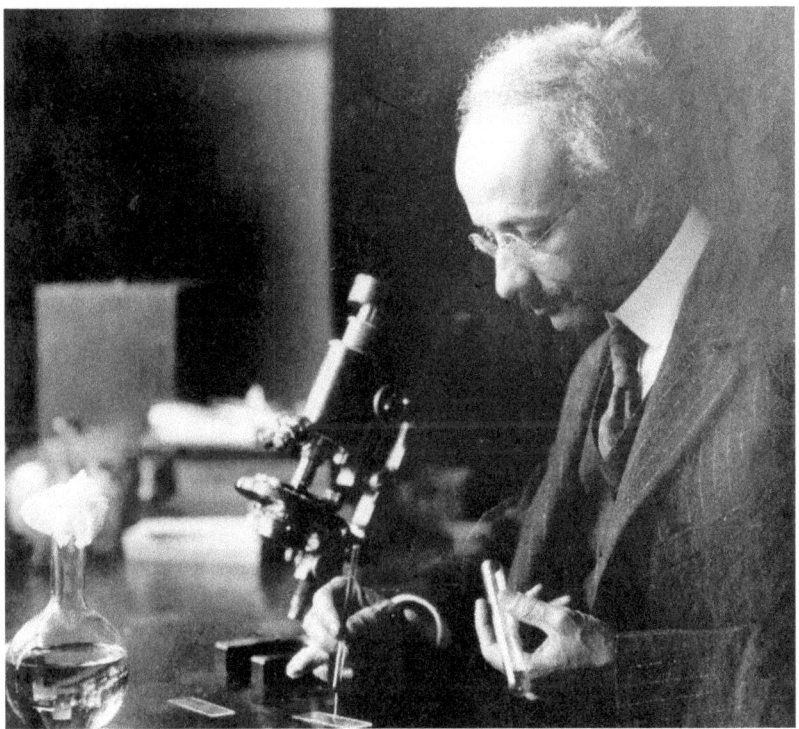

Solomon Carter Fuller, date unknown (Boston University Alumni Medical Library Archives).

The Boston Psychopathic Hospital

Arrangements were made for the trainees to work as volunteer interns at the Boston Psychopathic Hospital under the director of Dr. Campbell. The first private hospital for the insane in Massachusetts, the Boston Psychopathic Hospital admitted its first patient on October 6, 1818. Renamed the McLean Asylum in 1826 for John McLean who had bequeathed a large sum of money, the building was situated on the grounds of a former estate overlooking a small stream called Miller's River in the Charlestown area of Boston. Its name changed back to Boston Psychopathic Hospital, became part of the Boston State Hospital and was relocated to Fernwood Road, a five-minute walk from Harvard Medical School.

The Tuskegee Veterans Hospital and Its Black Physicians

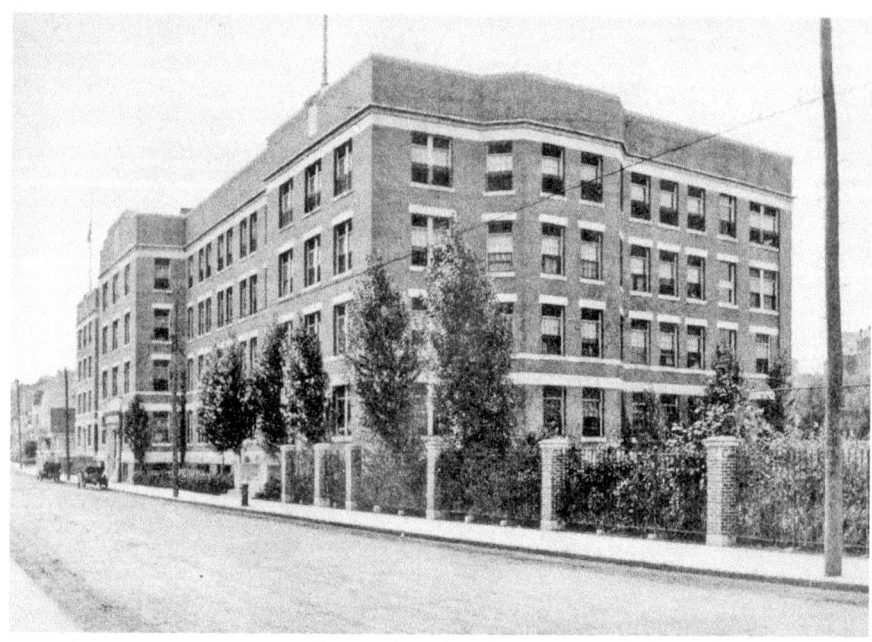

Boston Psychopathic Hospital, 74 Fernwood Road (*History of the Psychopathic Hospital* [Boston: Wright & Potter Printing Company, 1922]).

With the passage of legislation in 1910 titled "An Act Relative to Persons Suffering From Certain Mental Disorders who are Arrested or Confined in the City of Boston," the hospital was mandated to provide temporary observation, medical care and treatment to persons suffering from delirium, mania, mental confusion, delusions, or hallucinations who were arrested or came under the care or protection of the police of the city of Boston.[14]

While attending Boston University Medical School, Dr. Fuller had been inspired by Dr. Elmer Southard, one of his teachers and the first director of the Psychopathic Department at Boston Psychopathic Hospital. It was Dr. Southard who had encouraged Fuller to study neuropathology, a relative newcomer to medical science. Remembered by Fuller as "a great teacher, a great histologist," Southard was instrumental in establishing for the first time in the history of psychiatry, the cause of a mental disease (syphilitic psychoses) as well as a specific drug to treat the disease.[15] Under the direction of Dr. Southard, the

3. Black Physicians at the Tuskegee Hospital

hospital developed a reputation as a center for psychiatric investigation and training.[16] He and his staff made significant contributions to such areas of neuropsychiatric research as encephalitis, meningitis, epilepsy, and anaphylaxis.

Boston Psychopathic Hospital offered a unique opportunity for training that combined the medical specialties of neurology and psychiatry. In 1914, an important step in the training of physicians was

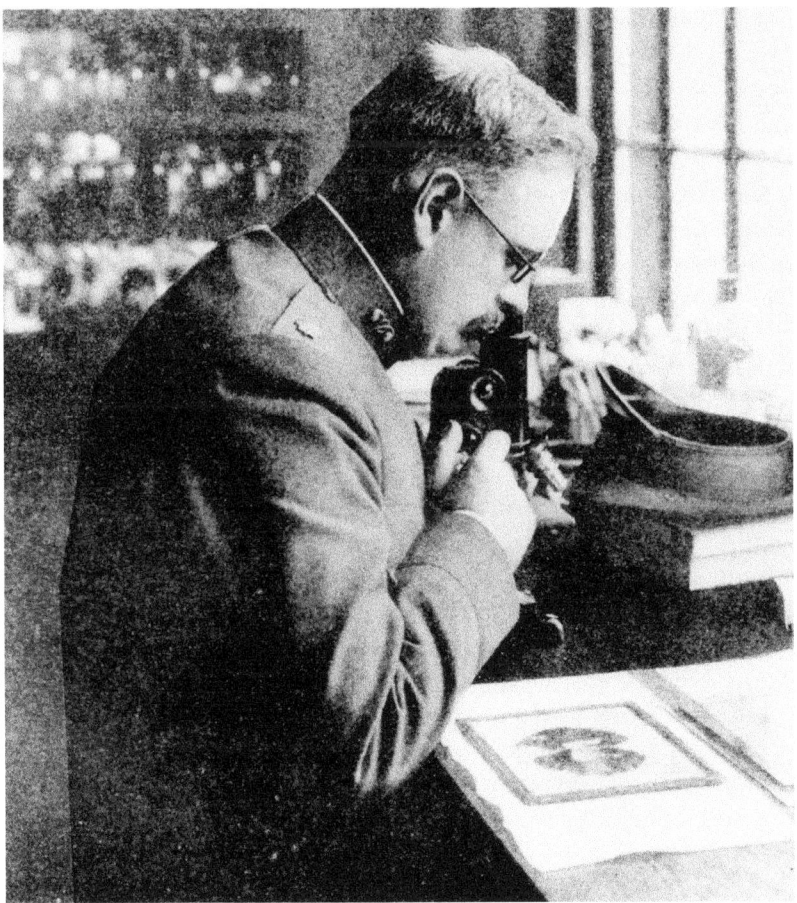

Major Elmer E. Southard, director of the training course conducted at the Boston Psychopathic Hospital for the U.S. army (*History of the Psychopathic Hospital* [Boston: Wright & Potter Printing Company, 1922]).

The Tuskegee Veterans Hospital and Its Black Physicians

taken by the Massachusetts Board of Insanity when it voted to require candidates for positions in any of the State hospitals to take a course of instruction in psychiatric hospital treatment.[17] Arrangements were made with Boston Psychopathic Hospital to offer special courses of from three to six months in order to qualify them for the positions. The courses were arranged to meet the specific needs of each trainee and included classes on admission of patients; clinical history-taking; insanity laws; intelligence tests (Binet-Simon, Yerkes, etc.); general mental examinations; methods of laboratory diagnosis of organic disease; principles of the Wassermann method; colloidal gold test; and cytology of cerebrospinal fluid. The trainees were given the title intern and received training, as well as lodging, free of charge.

The hospital program was influenced by the success of the army's mental treatment program during World War I. The institution was chosen by the U.S. surgeon general as one of six for special instruction in military psychiatry. The Department of Neuropsychiatry, directed by Thomas W. Salmon, brought together for the first time neurologists and psychiatrists who had returned from the war with expertise in both fields after treating soldiers' mental as well as physical wounds. In 1918, the hospital, in partnership with Smith College School of Social Work, developed a training program for the treatment of shell shock in returning veterans.[18]

The teaching was managed by the clinics and consisted of hospital lectures and actual ward experience.[19] Fuller's trainees also had the advantage of the learning opportunities provided by the hospital's clinical laboratory units that were just off the wards. There were special laboratories for bacteriology, chemistry, spinal fluid testing and histology as well as a research laboratory for metabolic studies. The hospital was known for its work on syphilis and the role that the disease plays in mental illness. Funding had been appropriated in 1912 to support the hospital's syphilis research and treatment program. As the number of patients entering the hospital and being seen at the outpatient clinic that were found to be suffering from syphilis increased, the scope of the syphilis program was expanded to include outpatient treatment of syphilitic patients. Various methods of treatment of general paresis were carried out and studied, including intensive intravenous arsphenamin therapy which was demonstrated to have beneficial

3. Black Physicians at the Tuskegee Hospital

effects on some of the patients. The experience and instruction provided to Fuller's trainees in the diagnosis and treatment of various types of syphilis would serve them well in their work at the veterans hospital. Most significant were the tools that enabled them to accurately diagnose black World War I veterans who had been diagnosed previously as having behavioral disorders and had been discharged from the military due to bad conduct, making them ineligible for veterans benefits.[20]

In November 1923, Drs. Toussaint T. Tildon, George Branche, Simon O. Johnson, and Harvey Davis completed their training and reported for duty at the Tuskegee Veterans Hospital. In later years, these men would recall not only Fuller's teaching but also the positive influence he had on their careers.

4

Fuller's Trainees

George Branche

Born on January 10, 1896, in Louisburg, North Carolina, George Branche was the youngest of six sons born to the Rev. Joel Branche and Hannah Shaw Branche. His mother died after giving birth to her twelfth child and he was raised by his maternal uncle and his wife. Although his grandparents were slaves during a time when they were not allowed to learn to read and write, his grandmother had encouraged her children to play school with the master's children so that they could learn. When slavery ended, all of her children became teachers.[1]

George attended the Mary Potter Academy, a Presbyterian school that was founded by his uncle, George Clayton Shaw, in the nearby town of Oxford. Dr. Shaw was one of the first black students to attend Princeton Theological Seminary, leaving the school after enduring a year of racist taunts. He received his degree from the Auburn Theological Seminary in New York and returned to his hometown in Oxford where he established the Timothy Darling Presbyterian Church in 1888. Concerned that there were no schools for African Americans in the area, he started the academy in 1889. The boarding school prepared students in normal and preparatory courses, offering Latin and Greek. Both Dr. Shaw and his wife, Mary Elizabeth Lewis Shaw, who taught at the school, played important roles in the education of African Americans in the South.

After graduating from high school in 1913, George entered Lincoln University in southern Chester County, Pennsylvania. Founded as the Ashmun Institute in 1854, the school was renamed Lincoln University in 1866 after the assassination of President Abraham Lincoln.[2] The

4. Fuller's Trainees

first degree-granting historically black university in the United States established for the collegiate and theological education of men, its graduates accounted for 20 percent of African American physicians from 1854 to 1954. Most of the students came from well-to-do families who were able to afford the school's high tuition, in addition to room and board, and who placed high expectations on their sons to succeed academically and professionally.

In addition to its emphasis on liberal arts education, Lincoln's sports teams dominated the black sports world. George played basketball and tennis, a sport that was generally not open to African Americans during that time. His grandson, George C. Branche III, recalls that this love for the game of tennis was passed down through the generations. A member of his high school varsity tennis team, George III has been the tournament physician for the Legg Mason Tennis Classic and the physician for several high school athletic teams.[3]

Following his graduation from Lincoln University in 1917, George was admitted to the Boston University School of Medicine. George C. Branche III has his grandfather's copy of the anatomy textbook that he used in medical school and says that their family had instilled a tradition of the value of education. George's two sons also graduated from the Boston University School of Medicine, his grandson received his medical degree from Howard University, and his great-granddaughter, a premed student at St. Louis University, is continuing the tradition, becoming the fourth generation to pursue medicine.[4]

Harvey Davis

Harvey Franklin Davis was born on August 22, 1893, in Chase City, Virginia, the second youngest of ten children born to Cephas and Hennetta Davis.

Prior to entering Boston University School of Medicine, Harvey attended Howard University. In 1917, while a student at Howard, he enlisted in the military. His military registration papers indicate that he received an exemption from the draft for an unspecified physical disability, making it doubtful that he served in active duty.

The requirements for entering the medical school at that time were to have an undergraduate diploma or to have completed two years of collegiate work. Since the school has no record of an undergraduate degree received by Harvey Davis, it is assumed that he met the second standard and did not graduate from Howard.[5]

Simon Overton Johnson

Born in McIntosh, Georgia on December 1, 1895, Simon Overton Johnson was the son of Amon and Celia Johnson.

He received an A.B. from Biddle Memorial Institute in Charlotte, North Carolina, in 1918. The historically black college, established in 1867 and affiliated with the Presbyterian Church, was later renamed in memory of Johnson C. Smith, a Pittsburgh banker and railroad pioneer. Following his graduation, Simon enlisted in the military, serving for less than one year before entering the Boston University School of Medicine. In addition to his training under the supervision of Dr. Fuller at the Boston Psychopathic Hospital, Simon also studied at Montefiore Hospital in New York, in Paris at Salpetiere Hospital, and at the National Hospital in London.[6]

Toussaint Tildon

Toussaint Tildon was born on April 5, 1893, in Waxahachie, Texas. He was the youngest son of three children born to John Wesley and Margaret Hilburn Tildon. His father was a teacher and principal of the Negro High School in Waxahackie who later earned his medical degree at the Chicago Medical College and returned to Texas to practice medicine. Having earned his undergraduate degree at Lincoln University in Pennsylvania, John Wesley Tildon was instrumental in sending many African American high school graduates from Texas to his alma mater. For those who were unable to afford the tuition, he often helped to defray their expenses or helped them obtain scholarships.[7]

Toussaint Tildon entered Lincoln University at the age of 15, receiving his bachelor's degree in 1912. His father had hoped that he would become a physician and sent him to Harvard to enroll in a

4. Fuller's Trainees

preparatory course for medicine. Instead, Toussaint took a course in public speaking with the intent of going to law school. Disappointed, his father withdrew financial support and Toussaint left after a year. After several years of teaching in Brunswick, Georgia for the meager salary of $40 a month, he realized that he would not be able to save for law school and asked for his father's support to attend medical school. Toussaint entered Meharry Medical College in Nashville, Tennessee, where his brother had graduated, and a year later, he transferred to Harvard.

The only African American student enrolled at the Harvard University Medical School, Toussaint had started the program several months after the violent race riots that occurred during the "Red Summer of 1919" protesting the lynchings in the South and the segregation imposed by Jim Crow laws.[8] Boston had experienced its own riots and protests in 1915 after the showing of *Birth of a Nation*, a racist film that featured the Klan as heroes and Southern blacks as villains with a focus on the need to suppress blacks in order to protect white society.

The unfriendly racial climate at Harvard had intensified following a directive issued one year earlier by University President Abbott Lawrence Lowell, which banned blacks from the freshman dormitories and suggested limiting the number of Jewish students to fifteen percent of the student body. "Harvard University, scarcely having recovered its calm and self-satisfaction following the flurry over the admission of Jewish students, was called upon to fact another charge today that Negroes were barred from her million dollar freshman dormitories. 'Harvard is turning into a southern institution. The colored man is not wanted, and every distinction that can be made to make us drop out is being made,' declared George McKinnow, a prominent member of the Nile Club, today."[9]

Toussaint received his medical degree from Harvard in 1923, specializing in psychiatry and neurology.

Boston

The city of Boston provided a wealth of educational opportunities and experiences for the four medical students. The New England

The Tuskegee Veterans Hospital and Its Black Physicians

medical community had a strong tradition of medical psychotherapy. The social and intellectual history of New England that were part of the liberal secular trends in the age of reform, along with liberal religious and political movements, made the city a center in the United States for reforms in the treatment of the mentally ill and the development of the new field of psychoanalysis. With the new emphasis on scientific psychology as an academic discipline and the interaction with European psychiatry, the Boston area became the home of many leading psychiatrists, including G. Stanley Hall, Adolf Meyer, and William James. Sigmund Freud made his only visit to the United States in 1909 to lecture at Clark University's twentieth anniversary celebration, accompanied by Carl Jung from Zurich and Sandor Ferenczi from Budapest.

Within the New England medical community, interaction with European psychiatry, a tradition of medical psychotherapy, respect for new and differing medical viewpoints, and a growing interest in neurology created an exceptional learning environment for Fuller's trainees.

5

The Practice of Medicine by Black Physicians in the Jim Crow South

The rural landscape of Tuskegee was a world away from the urban environment of Boston. The hospital sat on just over 400 acres, approximately one and one-half miles outside of the town and one mile from Tuskegee Institute, encircled by ravines and swamps and dotted with shacks. Located forty miles southeast of Montgomery, in Macon County, the land surrounding the town was hilly, eroded, and its soil depleted by decades of planting cotton. Prior to the Civil War, the town of Tuskegee, situated in the region known as the "black belt" named for the richness of its black soil, had been a flourishing center of cotton growing in Alabama. In later years, the town became known for the Tuskegee Institute.

At the turn of the century, its founder, Booker T. Washington, had been successful at making connections with wealthy white philanthropists such as steel magnate Andrew Carnegie, railroad executive William H. Baldwin, and Sears & Roebuck president Julius Rosenwald. With the school's growing endowment, he had been able to build a large campus with well-respected faculty. In 1911, the college established the John Andrew Hospital, which became a major center for black physicians. Although the campuses of the veterans hospital, the John Andrew Hospital, and the Tuskegee Institute offered an intellectual environment for black professionals, the town of Tuskegee and the surrounding area was extremely segregated. Within walking distance of the three institutions were several thousand African Americans living in poverty.

The Tuskegee Veterans Hospital and Its Black Physicians

After the Civil War, the large slave-holding plantations were broken up into smaller tracts and were cultivated by tenant farmers. Remnants of slavery and plantation life continued to exist on the tenant farms, where tenants' children were kept out of school to work in the fields and corporal punishment was administered. Farm laborers' wages averaged fifty to seventy-five cents a day. The practice of giving clothing and supplies on credit, known as "furnishing," was taken out of the tenants' wages during the harvest, leaving them forever in debt.[1]

The area's rural black population was, for the most part, illiterate and in poor health, with a high incidence of syphilis, gonorrhea, malaria, pellagra, tuberculosis and malnutrition. They experienced a high death rate and infant mortality that was due to the large number of women infected with syphilis and suffering from malnutrition. They lived in houses that were built right on the ground—poorly built shacks with wooden shingle roofs that usually leaked. The houses had no plumbing and fireplaces provided their heat and cooking facilities. Windows had no panes or screens, only wooden shutters. Furnishings were meager and walls were often covered with the pictorial sections of newspapers.

Segregation was the accepted order of the day. Jim Crow legal statutes regulated almost all aspects of black life throughout the Southern states. These statutes dictated where blacks could eat, which seats they could occupy in theaters and on buses and trains, which jobs they could perform, where they could live, which water fountain and public toilet they could use, and which beaches and parks they could visit.[2] Blacks could not be addressed as "Mister" or "Miss." They were forced to enter white homes though back doors and ate their meals outside. Every black man who was beaten or lynched was, in the minds of many Southerners, a bad Negro who deserved his punishment. White men who took the law into their own hands were considered upholders of racial superiority and protectors of Southern women. Especially dangerous to the white man's laws were educated blacks. Frederick Douglass said: "The resistance is not to the colored man as a slave, a servant, or a menial. It is aimed at the Negro as a man.... It is only when he acquires education, property and influence, only when he attempts to rise and be a man among men that he invites repression. It is not to the Negro but the quality of the Negro that disturbs popular prejudice."[3]

5. Black Physicians in the Jim Crow South

In the town of Tuskegee, the danger of success was also acknowledged by black residents. Ned Cobb, an Alabama sharecropper, said:

> They didn't like to see a nigger with too much; ... and it caused 'em to throw a slang word about a "nigger" having all this, that, and the other.... The idea—"keep the dollar out the niggers' hands"—these white folks went rock bottom with that.... The white people was afraid the money would make the nigger act too much like his own man.... [My father] had money but—whenever the colored man prospered too fast, they worked every figure to cut your britches off you. So, to his way of thinking it weren't no use in climbing too fast ... if they was going to take everything you worked for when you got too high.[4]

Despite the ubiquity of Southern racism, the Tuskegee Veterans Hospital offered one of the best locations available to black physicians at that time in which to practice medicine and was one of the few hospitals in the country where they could receive training in surgery. Although Southern blacks suffered greatly from the effects of professional segregation, Northern blacks were not beyond the reach of this effect. The number of accredited internships available in black hospitals nationwide, virtually the only ones that accepted blacks, was 60 percent of the number of internships needed for the 120 new black medical school graduates.[5] Rather than accept a black physician, many white hospitals chose to leave internships unfilled. The opportunities were especially limited for black psychiatrists, who were restricted to working in the small number of black institutions and facilities and were not allowed to publish in mainstream professional journals.

Black physicians comprised a small, elite class, defined by education, wealth, and occupation, within the largely poverty-stricken and uneducated African American population in the South. The widespread belief that blacks were inferior to whites prevented them from being treated as equals in professional relationships. The black physician was excluded from practicing in white hospitals, which limited admitting privileges to members of local American Medical Association chapters.[6] Since no county professional organization in the South allowed blacks to join, they were unable to admit their patients for treatment. Black physicians had little, if any relationships with local and state health departments, which were under the control of white medical associations.

The Tuskegee Veterans Hospital and Its Black Physicians

The racism that placed limits on the opportunities for the education of black physicians was also a factor in their exclusion from the postgraduate courses and fellowships that provided continuing education. The inability to gain specialty training which was a requirement for board certification, was a significant factor in limiting the number of black physicians in the specialty practices that brought greater wealth and status. State and county health departments sponsored clinics for black physicians, but their focus was primarily on public health issues such as tuberculosis, venereal disease and sanitation.

In order to provide access to postgraduate education, several local and national black medical societies began to include continuing education at their annual meetings and conventions.

One of the best known seminars for black physicians, the John A. Andrews Clinic, was held annually at the hospital of the same name in Tuskegee. The one-day clinic was begun in 1912 in conjunction with the fourteenth annual meeting of the National Medical Association. John Kenney, the hospital's director and Booker T. Washington's personal physician, established the clinic, which was taught by many well-known leaders in black medicine, such as Daniel Hale Williams, Matthew Walker, and Charles Drew. The success of the clinic led to its expansion to three days, during which doctors from across Alabama and Georgia donated their services, providing free treatment to those unable to pay. The rural population throughout the region was invited to take advantage of a rare opportunity—to be treated by doctors of their own race. The black citizens in Tuskegee were supportive of the clinics, providing housing, food and a warm welcome to the visitors. The "Tuskegee spirit" was described by Dr. Kenney as a combination of love of humanity, support for community, and dedication to the common cause that bound the community together.[7] Segregation gave them their *raison d'etre*, and it was a reminder of the work still to be done, with Tuskegee at the forefront of this effort.

The John A. Andrews Clinical Society held its first postgraduate course in 1921 in Tuskegee. Attended by 126 physicians from across the country, the four-week program featured lectures and demonstrations by fifty-three physicians, thirty of whom were white.[8]

Like the rest of the African American population living in the Jim Crow South, the black physician learned not to antagonize the white

5. Black Physicians in the Jim Crow South

establishment. In order to achieve and maintain the social and financial success that their education and training enabled them to enjoy, they had to preserve their relationships with white physicians and not step outside agreed upon roles.[9] Their tacit acceptance of elements of Jim Crow society were indications of distinct class divisions within black communities in the South.

Many black physicians had achieved wealth and prominence in their community as a result of cultivating relationships with influential whites. They understood that much of their success had to do with maintaining the segregated system within the networks of hospitals and businesses. Therefore, the majority avoided any involvement with Civil Rights activities. Speaking in a manner that implied accommodation while concealing their true feelings and motivation was a tactic often used by black Southerners in an attempt to maintain the image of the "contented Negro." Henry Hooten of Tuskegee observed, "Most times we would use strategy rather than use force. Be very kind. Use psychology on them. That would be the first thing the white man thought you knew less about was psychology."[10]

While many African Americans saw a medical degree as a ticket out of the poverty and segregation of the South, Fuller's trainees saw an opportunity to return to the South to use their training to provide health care to a previously underserved population. A staff position at the country's first government hospital built to treat black veterans would allow them to practice medicine and engage in research at a time when black physicians were denied hospital admitting privileges and staff positions at public hospitals in the Jim Crow South.

There were three patterns of providing hospital services to black patients in the South. The all-black hospital was built exclusively for black patients. The physicians and nurses in many of these hospitals were white, in others, they were biracial or black. The mixed-race hospitals were of two types. Most of them segregated blacks in separate wards, usually in all-black wings, basements, or attics. The other type was a facility with separate building attached to the main hospital, or separate building located on the hospital grounds. Generally, in mixed-race hospitals, only white physicians and nurses were admitted to the professional staffs. In some cases, black physicians continued to care for their hospitalized patients, but were only allowed in the black

The Tuskegee Veterans Hospital and Its Black Physicians

wards. In all-white hospitals, which were the majority in the South, blacks were refused admission in all but the most extreme emergency situations.[11]

Fuller's trainees soon found that as black physicians living in the segregated South, they were considered an elite class in their community. While they were very much a part of the black community, they were significantly different from most blacks in Tuskegee due to their education, occupation and wealth. George Branche's son George remembers growing up on the grounds of the Tuskegee hospital and how much that rarified environment protected him, his brother, Matt, his sister, Martie, and the other children of the medical staff from the very segregated world of the Tuskegee community outside the hospital gates. "There were several Tuskegee families who lived on the grounds in an area we called 'the circle,' and they were all doctors tied to the Hospital. We were protected from the bigotry of the town in so many ways. We went to an elementary school on the grounds and had a swimming pool and tennis courts there as well. We also grew up seeing many famous black people like George Washington Carver and General Benjamin Davis and others."[12]

Because of their concern about the quality of the schools in the South, many of the physicians sent their children to the Children's House, a school situated on the Tuskegee Institute campus. It was also not uncommon for the families to send their children to the North for their higher education. In a 2001 interview, Branche's daughter, Martie, described her family's plan to obtain quality education for their three children.

> Father was concerned that his children receive a better education. Mother had been a schoolteacher. Decided that they wanted the children to go to school in Boston. Since her father could not leave his job in Tuskegee, her parents made a supreme sacrifice and established two households. Mother took the children to Boston when Martie was about 7 years old. Father came when he could for visits. Every summer the family reunited in Tuskegee. In Boston [they] lived in a brownstone which contained three large apartments. All the apartments were occupied by her large extended family, which included close friends and godparents. The Branche family occupied the second story of this brownstone, which was a 71 Highland Street, until she graduated from high school. Brothers continued to live there after school while they attended medical schools. Wartime limited travel to Tuskegee. Army took over the medical corps and VA

5. Black Physicians in the Jim Crow South

doctors, so her father got some additional travel privileges because he was now in the army.[13]

After graduating from the Dillaway Elementary School for Girls, Martie Branche completed her studies at the Girls' Latin School and then went on to Sarah Lawrence College and graduate school at Columbia University where she received a Masters in Psychiatric Social Work.

Dr. Branche's sons, George, Jr., and Archon Matthew, also attended the Boston Latin School. They received their undergraduate degrees at Bowdoin College and graduated from the Boston University Medical School.

Dr. Tildon's three children were also educated in Northern schools. His two sons, Toussaint Jr. and John Wesley, one of his daughters, Helen Hortense, and a grandson all became physicians. Toussaint Jr., who received his undergraduate degree at Amherst College and his M.D. at Howard University, would return to Tuskegee in the 1960s to become chief of thoracic and vascular surgery and to develop a residency training program in the diagnostic and therapeutic aspects of these specialties.

Harvey F. Davis, Jr., also followed in the footsteps of his father and chose a career in medicine. He became a nurse, earning his R.N. degree and a Ph.D., and worked at the Centers for Disease Control (CDC) in Atlanta, Georgia.

Toussaint Tildon's granddaughter, Margaret Calhoun Williams, who also grew up in Tuskegee, recalls that although she did not grow up on the hospital campus like her mother, she did not experience the town's racism in the way that others might have. As a child, she was a member of Jack and Jill, a non-profit service organization for children.[14] Established in 1938, the national organization, with chapters throughout the United States and Germany, was viewed by the black elite as a means by which to network with other members of the black professional class and to introduce their children to educational, social and cultural experiences. Like her mother and many of the children of the hospital's black medical staff, Margaret left Tuskegee in ninth grade to attend boarding school at Northfield Mount Herman in Massachusetts.

The black physicians who were on staff at the Tuskegee Veterans Hospital did not live or practice in a vacuum. They actively contributed

The Tuskegee Veterans Hospital and Its Black Physicians

to the civic development of the hospital, the community and their churches. Both Tildon and Branche were elders in their churches. But, like the rest of the black community, they were subject to some of the same social indignities and legal obstacles. They had to sit in the balcony of the movie theatre and drink from the "colored" water fountains.

6

The Tuskegee Veterans Hospital
Challenges, Successes and Scandal

The 1920s

Shortly after the four physicians completed their work in psychiatry at Boston University under Dr. Fuller and arrived in Tuskegee, the veterans hospital was placed under the management of its first black administrator, Dr. Joseph H. Ward. With the staffing of blacks at the hospital, the hope was that black veterans would be treated with respect and dignity in a caring environment, one that did not exist in most of the hospitals that admitted black patients. Dr. Ward, a graduate of the Indiana University School of Medicine, was a highly regarded physician who was vice president of the National Hospital Association. He had worked briefly at the prestigious Mayo Clinic in Rochester, Minnesota and had received training in several Veterans Bureau hospitals prior to being assigned to Tuskegee where he was initially appointed the Chief of Surgery. A World War I veteran who had served overseas as a major in the medical corps, and held the rank of lieutenant colonel at the time of his appointment, Dr. Ward shared his goals for the expansion of the hospital.[1] Dr. Ward wrote to Dr. Louis T. Wright, "My intention is to place this hospital on very high grounds. My first goal will be to lift it out of the class of an insane asylum or hospital, and I might add with force, to lift it out of the class of a Tuberculosis hospital, to that of a big General Hospital for our race. If I can succeed in doing that, I will feel that I have accomplished something along our line."[2]

Soon after Dr. Ward assumed the leadership of the hospital, there were rumors of internal discord among some of the black administrative staff. Charges and counter-charges reached a head in June 1925 when W. L. Jones, chief engineer, filed a number of charges against Dr. Ward's administration with the Veterans Bureau. These charges included serving a luncheon for the black physicians who attended the annual Tuskegee Institute Clinic held in April of that year; the erection of garages for the use of physicians on the staff; the use of gas in Dr. Ward's private car; the use of hospital trucks to haul musical instruments and trunks from Chehaw to Tuskegee for musical entertainment; sharing of the water supply with Tuskegee Institute; and being dominated by Dr. Moton, president of Tuskegee Institute. Upon investigation of the charges, it was discovered that Mr. Jones, with the aid of others in his conspiracy, had "planted" one of his men in Dr. Ward's office as an orderly. He was able to obtain information which he distorted and used in the effort to destroy Dr. Ward. The charges were proven to be false and Jones was suspended from duty at the hospital.

Instead of leaving town, Jones remained in the community and continued to collect information about hospital affairs through his co-conspirators who remained employed at the facility. Anonymous letters and forged affidavits were sent to the Veterans Administration Bureau, creating a situation in which Dr. Ward was forced to be constantly defending himself. Through an investigation by Melvin Chisum, field secretary for the National Negro Press Association, it was determined that Mr. Jones was involved in a conspiracy with Dr. Nelson, a Tuskegee physician who had previously been jailed for misappropriating funds for the building of a general hospital in the town.[3]

Known for his fairness in dealing with hospital personnel and his fearlessness in working with community groups, Dr. Ward acquired an enviable reputation in the Tuskegee community. His inspection tours on horseback were legendary. He remained in charge of the hospital until 1936 when Dr. Eugene H. Dibble, Jr., who was serving as medical director of the John A. Andrew Hospital, was appointed to his position.

6. The Tuskegee Veterans Hospital

While it was expected that Fuller's trainees would assume their positions in the hospital's psychiatric section, Dr. Branche was soon transferred from psychiatry to the medical service because of a critical shortage of physicians at the hospital. A year later, he was selected to serve as the acting chief of neuropsychiatric service for five months pending the arrival of Dr. George Moore. Branche took a one-year leave from the hospital in 1927, when he completed an internship in general medicine at Kansas City General Hospital in Missouri. Upon his return, he was promoted to associate medical officer in the surgical service.

Harvey Davis was another of Dr. Fuller's trainees whose career path at the Tuskegee hospital took a different direction. World War I was the first war in which a large number of combat victims survived. Many of the veterans returned with amputations, reduced lung capacity from being gassed, head injuries, and "shell shock." A new service was being developed to rehabilitate these veterans and Davis was instrumental in establishing a program at the Tuskegee facility.

On June 25, 1927, a separate building was dedicated on hospital grounds for patient rehabilitation and recreation.[4] Following the programs of Canada and England, the rehabilitation of hospital patients focused on teaching them skills in trades such as shoemaking, tailoring, typing, stenography, and telegraphy. Training in agricultural industries, such as farming, was also provided. Recreation activities were also available to the veterans. Although recreation facilities for veterans had been established in communities throughout the country, most were segregated and not available for black soldiers in the South.[5]

It wasn't long before Fuller's trainees were joined by other highly qualified black physicians as members of the hospital staff during this period, Dr. Eugene Dibble, Jr., a graduate of Howard Medical School in 1919, became chief of the surgery department in 1924. He had interned at the John A. Andrew Hospital at Tuskegee Institute and at the time of his appointment was in private practice. Dr. Dibble remained only a short time, before leaving to become director of the John A. Andrew Hospital. He later returned to the VA as its manager in 1936.

Dr. George S. Moore, a former professor of nervous and mental diseases at Meharry Medical College, was appointed clinical director

The Tuskegee Veterans Hospital and Its Black Physicians

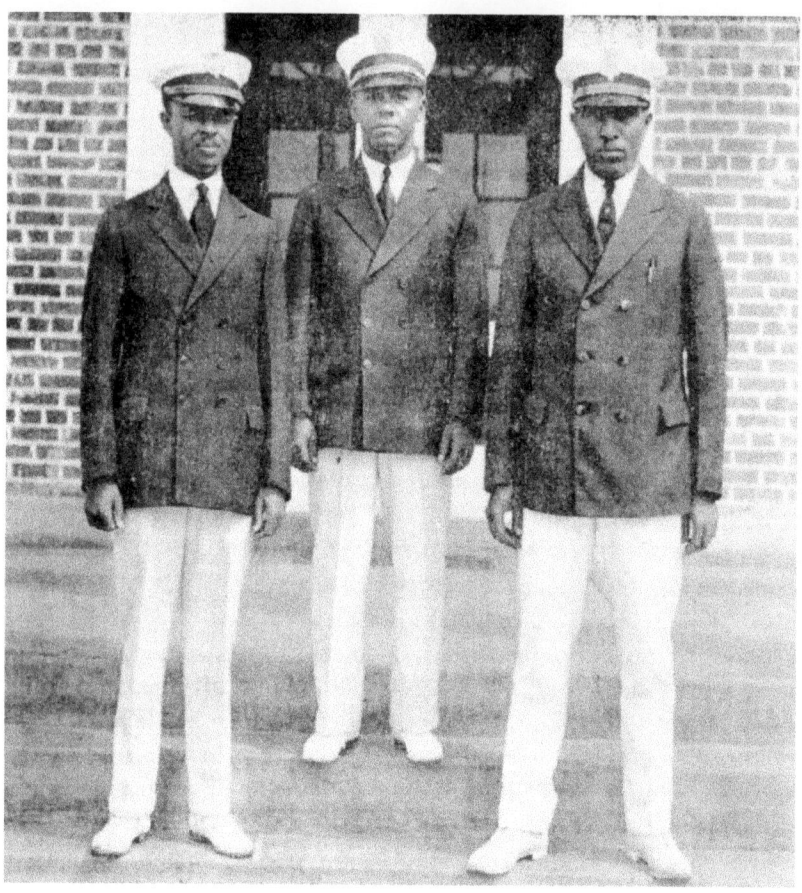

Left to right, Drs. Tildon, Davis, and Branche at the dedication of the recreation building, U.S. Veterans Hospital, June 25, 1927 (Tuskegee University Archives, Tuskegee, Alabama).

of psychiatry. Respected as an intuitive clinician with an understanding of the influence of cultural factors in psychoses in black patients, he published two articles in the Veterans Bureau medical bulletin entitled *An Introduction to a Study of Neuropsychiatric Problems Among Negroes*.[6] In the articles, he pointed out that a psychiatrist could not make an accurate diagnosis without knowledge of black psychology and might misdiagnose mental deficiency based on feigned cultural ignorance and tests that were not validated for blacks. He also warned of a potential

6. The Tuskegee Veterans Hospital

misdiagnosis of paranoid psychosis made as a result of a reaction to a hostile environment.

In 1925, Dr. William Fletcher Penn assumed responsibility as chief of surgery, a position he held until his death in 1934. Penn was a graduate of Yale University Medical School, where he held the distinction of being the school's first African American student. On completing an internship at Freedmen's Hospital in Washington, D.C., he returned to his hometown of Atlanta and opened a medical and surgical practice. While in Atlanta, he established Mercy Hospital and served as its superintendent and chief of the surgical service for many years before coming to Tuskegee. He had a reputation as the leading physician in south Atlanta, caring for both white and black patients and conducting surgical clinics to help his colleagues advance their skills.

Dr. John A. Kenney, the medical director of the John A. Andrew Hospital who had fled Tuskegee after being threatened by the Klan when the veterans hospital opened, returned after a two-month stay in the North. He remained until 1924 when he resigned his position and left for Newark, New Jersey, to enter private practice. In 1927, he opened Kenney Memorial Hospital to provide medical care to Newark's black population. Dr. Kenney would return to Tuskegee in 1939 to take over the administration of the John A. Andrew Hospital. He was the president of the National Medical Association from 1904 until 1912, during which time he founded the association's journal. Dr. Kenney's son, Howard Washington Kenney, would later return to Tuskegee where he served as medical director of both the John A. Andrew Hospital and the VA hospital.

Dr. Drue King, a graduate of Tufts Medical College, had come to Tuskegee for an internship at the John A. Andrew Hospital in the fall of 1914. He resigned from his position as an intern on February 14, 1915, following a reprimand by Dr. Kenney, the medical director. Kenney wrote to Booker T. Washington:

> I called him to the office to speak to him about it. His whole manner and attitude with reference to the matter was unsatisfactory. I told him that we were not accustomed to such language in our hospital. He remarked that perhaps I had never had a Northern man before. I asked him if he used this language generally. He said that he did not know, that he had not thought about it and had spoken in a plain, natural way.

The Tuskegee Veterans Hospital and Its Black Physicians

> In this connection I also had to speak to him about conducting a lady teacher into the internes' bed room to see one of the internes who was sick. Even tho [sic] the matron states positively that she saw him take the lady in the room, he denies it, but said in connection with it that if he did do it, what of it? That they were men and not students and if he wanted a lady carried in it was his privilege and that he did not wish any further discussion about it and if I wished to say anything else about it I could say it to you.[7]

After several years of private practice in Augusta, Georgia, King returned to Tuskegee to accept a position at the VA. Drue King suffered a cerebral hemorrhage and died while at work at the VA on April 20, 1947. His death certificate is signed by George Branche.

By the end of the 1920s, the veterans hospital was staffed completely by black doctors of the highest quality. In general operative efficiency, the facility ranked above average according to statements made by Veterans Bureau officials, the National Negro Press Association, and other respected medical professionals. "It was expected that in the conduct of so large an enterprise without previous experience in handling a gigantic government institution, the Negro personnel would make some mistakes, but it is surprising that their mistakes have been so few."[8] Dr. Louis T. Wright wrote in *The Crisis*: "I am told that this hospital has been rated since it was first established as one of the best managed Veterans Hospitals in the country, both as to administration and in the character of scientific work done."[9] Dr. Joseph Garland, of Massachusetts General Hospital, said, "The Tuskegee Veterans' Hospital is one of the best conducted. The two hospitals at Tuskegee probably comprise the most fertile field for clinical material that the Negro race possess."[10]

In 1929, it was reported that the hospital was operating at almost full capacity of 609 patients, with a daily average of 550. The number of employees totaled 344, comprised of twenty-three physicians, two dentists, one pharmacist, three laboratory technicians, three physiotherapy aides, seven occupational therapy aides, two librarians, four dieticians, and fifty-two nurses.[11]

The hospital was engaged in state-of-the-art medical care that included the successful use of deep x-ray therapy; successful liver treatment in pernicious anemia; the treatment of general paresis by malaria inoculation; and the use of ventricolography for the roentgen diagnosis

6. The Tuskegee Veterans Hospital

of intracranial conditions. Autopsies showed an error in diagnoses of less than five percent. In order to advance the medical knowledge of the staff, Dr. Ward established a medical society that held regular meetings where doctors presented papers on special topics and cases.

It was the general opinion that Dr. Ward had measured up to the responsibilities of his position. The first few years of internal dissent and conspiracy and the lack of confidence of the public had made his job difficult, but his ability to build a well-qualified and cooperative staff gained him respect and brought recognition to the hospital.

The 1930s

In 1930, the State Board of Health of Alabama reported that fifty-four counties serving 88 percent of the state's population were participating in the state health program. Each county had a county health officer and at least one nurse. Public health specialists from other states came to study the Alabama Health Department organization, which was now considered a model program.[12]

In 1938, the South had been identified as "the Nation's No. 1 health problem" by Surgeon General Thomas Parran, based on such regional disparities as shorter life spans and fewer physicians and hospital beds.[13] With the help of the NAACP, in addition to both African American and white reformers, the U.S. Public Health pushed for federal funds to improve the health of Southerners. The Hill-Burton Act of 1946 (officially known as the Hospital Survey and Construction Act) would later be enacted as a result of Jim Crow policy. The act established need-based fund allocation for hospital construction and was the first major federal legislation in the twentieth century to include a non-discrimination clause. In granting funds for the construction and expansion of biracial hospitals, Hill-Burton increased the access of both African American and white patients to hospital care in the South.[14]

In August 1931, the National Medical Association and the National Hospital Association proposed the establishment of a second black veterans hospital. Racial discrimination continued to limit black access to most veterans hospitals, with many receiving care in segregated wards. The organizations also contended that the additional hospital would provide more opportunities for black professionals. The number of internships available for black medical school graduates continued to be small. For the 122 blacks who graduated in 1932, there were only 110 internships in comparison to more than 6000 internships available for the 4,814 white medical graduates. Of 354 hospitals approved for medical residencies, only three would accept blacks. There were no residencies for blacks in tuberculosis, orthopedics, and pediatrics.[15]

The proposal was criticized by the NAACP, which considered it the "height of irony to set apart veterans wounded in a war for democracy in hospitals where such separation is based on skin color."[16] NAACP president Walter White argued that the existence of the Tuskegee Hospital had hampered efforts to integrate all veterans hospitals and that black veterans were often denied admission to hospitals closer to their homes and transferred to Tuskegee. He also criticized the NMA's support of separate, tax-supported facilities because he viewed them as a form of government-sponsored segregation. When a bill was introduced by Republican senator David Reed of Pennsylvania to build a black veterans hospital in the North, at the request of the American Legion, both medical organizations and the NAACP opposed it, and a second hospital for black veterans was never built.

The training in syphilis that his trainees received from Dr. Solomon Carter Fuller and at the Boston Psychopathic Hospital proved to be invaluable in their work at the Tuskegee VA. The venereal disease rate among black soldiers was almost three times as high as among white troops and very few of them had received any medical treatment beyond taking a patent medicine, sometimes referred to as "snake oil," which was ineffective.[17]

A large group of the hospital's patients suffered from syphilis of the brain and spinal cord and were unable to be treated by the then acceptable method of malaria therapy. Black patients did not respond to the tertian strain of malaria fever, which was then in use.[18] In 1932, after several years of research, Dr. George Branche, who had been promoted to assistant clinical director, developed a new method of treatment. He found that by the use of the quartan strain of malaria, which was a foreign strain to which the black patient had not developed an immunity, beneficial results were seen. Dr. Branche published the results

6. The Tuskegee Veterans Hospital

of his research in a series of articles in which he reported that more than 500 cases had been treated, with a large number of complete recoveries and returns to employment.

With the effectiveness of this strain of malaria established, the Tuskegee hospital was able to furnish blood to other Veterans Administration facilities and to many state institutions. The development of the quartan strain of malaria was seen as an important contribution in the treatment of neurosyphilis in the African American population.[19] This difference in biological therapy—"white people respond best to tertian malaria, Negroes to quartan"—was acknowledged in both the syphilology and malariology literature.[20]

Dr. Eugene H. Dibble was appointed manager of the hospital in 1936, serving until 1946, when he returned to the John A. Andrew Hospital to become the medical director. He was given a directive to reorganize the hospital, which was facing a shortage of adequate numbers of medical and dental personnel. Dr. Tildon, who had been promoted to clinical director of medical services in 1937, often served as acting manager in Dr. Dibble's absence.

In 1939, Dr. Charles Prudhomme, a well-known physician in the Division of Neurology and Psychiatry at Howard University, accepted an assignment as associate medical officer at the hospital. In 1943, after about four and a half years in Tuskegee, he returned to Howard.

The Great Depression

With the arrival of the 1930s came the Great Depression. Like the majority of the nation's population, the black professional class also experienced economic losses. African Americans who had built successful medical practices were confronted with the same Depression-related problems as other physicians, but their hardships were even more acute because the patients that they provided care for were poorer. In Macon County, food advances to the tenants and sharecroppers were cut by landowners and merchants after crops were planted in the spring of 1931. Organizers were sent to Alabama by the Communist Party to build a sharecroppers union in the rural farm areas.[21]

The Tuskegee VA was an important source of employment for

blacks during this time of high unemployment. Many hospitals and clinics that had been established by black physicians were unable to survive the hardships of the Depression. Faced with a diminishing number of patients who could afford to pay for care and worsening health among blacks, some black physicians began encouraging their patients to demand admission to the segregated government-operated hospitals and clinics.[22]

There was little effort on the part of President Herbert Hoover to use the federal government to intervene in order to provide economic relief. While he did attempt to convince businesses to retain employees and not to cut wages, as well as approve loans to banks, railroads and insurance companies, he suggested that the needs of the unemployed and the homeless be met by local governments and charities. As a result, wandering groups of men, women and children began settling into squalid clusters of shacks made of tin, cardboard, and burlap adjacent to railroad tracks and dumps called "Hoovervilles."

The Tuskegee Study

For many scientists and scholars today, Tuskegee is best known as the site of one of the worst manifestations of racism in American society. There, in 1932, the U.S. Public Health Service began a study of syphilis, a sexually transmitted disease that, if untreated, can cause paralysis, dementia, and heart failure. The Alabama State Board of Health had begun a campaign against venereal disease in 1918 in response to war-related efforts of the federal government.[23] Initially a major component of a social hygiene program, syphilis became the focus of the state's health officials following the withdrawal of federal funds in 1919. In 1927, Alabama's state legislature passed legislation that required persons who were infected with venereal disease to report for treatment to a reputable physician and to continue treatment until the disease was no longer communicable or a source of danger to public health.[24]

Entitled "The Tuskegee Study of Untreated Syphilis in the Male Negro," the program recruited 622 black men in Macon County who were poor sharecroppers, many of them illiterate. Of those subjects,

6. The Tuskegee Veterans Hospital

431 had advanced cases of syphilis. The rest were free of the disease and served as the control group for comparison.[25] Macon County was selected as the project site based on a 1930 study of six Southern counties to determine the prevalence of syphilis in rural areas where blacks constituted a large percentage of the population. In the study, Macon County was found to have the highest percentage of syphilis, with 35 percent of the 3,363 blacks testing positive for the disease.[26]

When the project in Macon County was started, it was funded by grants from the Rosenwald Foundation and involved the setting up of twenty-nine clinics in churches, schools, the court house, and at the John Andrew Hospital. The project physicians would use their cars, carrying their equipment in them, and treat or give blood tests at the designated sites. Nurses carried kits for taking blood into homes in order to find cases. After several years, this method of case finding and treatment was found to be unsatisfactory because of poor conditions in the homes, such as inadequate water, heat, and facilities for examination and sterilization. A bus was then outfitted as a clinic, with running water, sterilizers, and examining rooms. Each day, the bus would travel to a designated area, eventually covering every rural section of Macon County.

The Rosenwald Fund withdrew its support for the program two years later because of financial difficulties during the Depression. The fund viewed long-term, comprehensive treatment programs as the responsibility of state and local agencies. With the loss of outside funding, the Public Health Service took over the project and what had originally been a treatment program, was now an experiment, designed to follow the development and progression of untreated syphilis. It would become the longest experiment in withholding treatment from human subjects in medical history, lasting for over thirty years.

The five survey periods in the study occurred in 1932, 1938–39, 1948, 1952–53, and 1968–70. The original study group was composed of 399 men who received no therapy and who had historical and laboratory evidence of syphilis which had progressed beyond the infectious stages, and 201 men comparable in age and environment who were determined to be free of syphilis that were selected to be in control group.[27]

The study was initiated by Public Health Service Surgeon General

The Tuskegee Veterans Hospital and Its Black Physicians

Hugh Cumming and directed by assistant surgeons general Taliaferro Clark and Raymond A. Vonderlehr during its first decade.[28] All three had graduated from medical school at the University of Virginia, a center of eugenics teaching, where students were taught that race was a key factor in the etiology and the natural history of syphilis.

The project was structured to compare an all-black cohort to an all-white sample analyzed in Norway in 1910, the only other study of untreated syphilis reported in the medical literature.[29]

The project was based on three assumptions that were rooted in the country's racist beliefs:

1. *The disease affected blacks differently than whites and thus was a legitimate focus of research.* While such ideas did not square well with the bulk of the medical evidence even at the time the study began in 1932, it continued to serve as the justification for a black only study.

This assumption was reinforced by Surgeon General Thomas Parran in 1937 when he wrote, "The Negro is not to blame because his syphilis rate is six times that of the white.... It is through no fault of hers that the colored woman remains infectious two and one-half times as long as the white woman."[30]

2. *Since the subjects had no access to medical care, whatever was provided was better than what they would have received without the project.* The subjects were "uncontaminated" by any form of treatment and thus more useful from a research perspective. They posed no ethical dilemma, at least from the perspective of the researchers, since they were not withholding something the subjects would have received in the absence of the experiment. When the project began, few of the subjects had ever seen a physician. Rural blacks in Alabama did not go to physicians. Thus, whatever care was provided to them, project directors argued, was better than what they would have received without participating in the project. Any questions asked about racial issues was to be handled by saying, "These people were getting better medical care than they would under any other circumstances."[31]

6. The Tuskegee Veterans Hospital

Through various public-health programs and eventually through the passage of Medicare and Medicaid, the availability of medical care for these subjects changed dramatically over the lifetime of the project.

3. *The subjects were poorly educated, poorly motivated, and the course of treatment was too demanding and complicated to assure the compliance necessary for success.* The treatment became less difficult and problematic with the introduction of antibiotics after World War II. Educational levels of the subjects and their families probably also increased. Yet the assumption that these rural Alabama black males were not good patients or good risks for treatment persisted.[32]

According to the final report issued by the Tuskegee Syphilis Study Ad Hoc Advisory Panel, the U.S. Department of Health, Education, and Welfare Public Health Service in 1973, there is no evidence that a written protocol ever existed that documented the original intent of the study.[33] It is assumed that the decision to continue the study as a long-term study was made in the first Annual Report of the Surgeon General for 1935–36, which included the statement, "Plans for the continuation of this study are underway. During the last 12 months, success has been obtained in gaining permission for the performance of autopsies on 11/15 individuals who died."

The panel also expressed the following concerns:

1. There was no evidence that informed consent was gained from the human subjects in the study;
2. There was evidence in 1932 that there were satisfactory outcomes in 85 percent of patients with latent syphilis that were treated in contrast to 35 percent if no treatment was given;
3. The description of the subjects as "untreated" was inaccurate. It was reported in 1946 that "about one-fourth of the syphilitic individuals received treatment for their infection." The "untreated" group in the study was therefore a group of treated and untreated male subjects. In a later report, it was stated that all but one of the originally untreated syphilitics seen in 1968–1970 had received therapy;

4. There was evidence that control subjects who became syphilitic were transferred from the "untreated" group. Since this transfer of patients from the control group did occur, the study is not one of late latent syphilis. It is also not certain that this group of patients did in fact receive therapy.

A letter dated November 28, 1938, from Dr. Austin V. Deibert, USPHS, to Dr. R. A. Vonderlehr, one of the study's directors, expresses concern about the increasing numbers of study participants who were in the "untreated syphilis" sample—40 percent, that had received some arsenical therapy. "In view of the following statements I acutely fear that adverse critism of the study would be justifiable, viewing it as an 'untreated group.'" In the letter, Dr. Deibert suggests supplementing the study with the plan to "(1) Maintain the syphilitic cases who have received some treatment as a study group of inadequately treated cases and on whom subsequent periodic observations can be made; and (2) Replace these cases with strictly new untreated men of comparable ages and infection dates."[34] In Dr. Vonderlehr's letter of response, dated December 5, 1938, he expresses surprise that Dr. Deibert was unaware of the treatment provided to study participants, indicating that he was under the impression that it had been discussed earlier. He justified the treatment by explaining that

> first, when the study was started in the fall of 1932, no plans had been made for its continuation and a few patients were treated before we fully realized the need for continuing the project on a permanent basis. Second, it was difficult to hold the interest of the group of Negroes in Macon County unless some treatment was given. This was particularly true in the patients with early syphilis. In consequence, we treated practically all of the patients with early manifestations and many of the patients with latent syphilis.... If it is not possible to add to the number of untreated syphilitic Negro males included in the study, it will, of course, be necessary to exclude all of those who were treated some years ago in the future. I doubt the wisdom of bothering to examine the treated individuals carefully because we already have in the clinics of the Cooperative Clinical Group a considerable number of Negro males in the proper age group who have received inadequate treatment and who are under observation.[35]

The panel's list of concerns continued:

5. In the absence of a definitive protocol, there was no evidence or assurance that standardization of evaluative procedures, which

6. The Tuskegee Veterans Hospital

are essential to the validity and reliability of a scientific study, existed at any time; and
6. There was absence of evidence that patients were given a "choice" of continuing in the study once penicillin became readily available.

In order to gain the trust of the participants, a black nurse, Eunice Rivers, was hired. She recruited the subjects by convincing them that they had "bad blood" and needed special treatment. The participants were monitored, receiving regularly scheduled physical examinations, which included a lumbar puncture, a procedure that involved the insertion of a needle into the spinal cord to obtain fluid for diagnosis. The study's physicians observed the subjects, keeping records of their health and performing autopsies on those who died. Benefits such as a regular physical examination, hot lunches provided on examination days, and a burial allowance were promoted to retain the study's subjects.

> What kind of people attend the clinic: Nearly all of the patients are farm laborers. Some of them are farm tenants; some—a few—own their own farms. Some of the patients are women. They are poorly dressed but as a rule are clean. Some may be dirty and they come to the clinic out of the fields, with dirt, bugs, and the odor of fertilizer on them. The shoes worn are very much worn out and too often one can see the toes of persons ticking out of the shoes, even in cold weather. Some don't wear any shoes. Most all kinds of shoes or would-be shoes are worn. Hats are scarce. Overalls are the principal mode of dress for the men.
>
> The homes of most of my patients are old, paintless, plasterless, poorly built shacks, with wooden shingle roofs, which leak when it rains and allow cold air and snow to enter in winter. It is unusual to find glass windows in those shacks. There open windows with a blind but no glass panes. There are open fireplaces for wood burning in all homes. This fireplace is used for heat as well as for cooking in some cases. Some homes have one room, some two rooms, few more rooms. The mother, father, 3, 4, 5, 6, 7 children stay in these rooms. As a rule there are two beds in the room. If Grandma is alive, she and Grandpa stay here also.[36]

While the general public was unaware of the Tuskegee experiment, black leaders and medical professionals in the community knew about the research study. Dr. George Washington Carver, whose research on the processing of peanut oil into metallic mercury to treat syphilis, was reported to have provided consultation and assistance to the study. The United States Public Health Service, state and county public health

The Tuskegee Veterans Hospital and Its Black Physicians

office and members of the local white medical society were all active participants.[37] Although the more than forty-year study was directed by white physicians, a number of black physicians were employed in the program, beginning with the initial medical survey of the incidence of syphilis in Macon County's African American population. H. L. Harris, Jr., the black physician hired by the Rosenwald Fund to conduct the survey, reported that it was "useless to attempt to cure syphilis in the Negro population in Macon County" until a comprehensive health program designed to "treat the large number of cases of tuberculosis, malnutrition and pellagra" was first implemented. Without a major health initiative for the county, he concluded, establishing any syphilis-control programs was useless. The comprehensive health program proposed by Dr. Harris was never initiated, but the results of his survey, indicating that 35 percent of the county's African American population was syphilitic, led the United States Public Health Service to propose the study of untreated syphilis.[38]

The question of how black physicians could participate in a program that used blacks as guinea pigs and denied them treatment has often been asked. It has been suggested that their involvement is an illustration of class divisions between black physicians and the larger black community and that the middle-class physicians did not identify with the study participants who were poor and uneducated. Their desire to prove to the white medical profession that they were capable of engaging in medical research may have also inspired them to support and take part in the syphilis study.

Outside professionals regularly reviewed the project's protocols. It also had the support and used the facilities of the VA hospital and the Tuskegee Institute. In 1937, United States Public Health Service officials approached Eugene Dibble, manager of the VA hospital, to request the use of the facility for the syphilis study.

February 9, 1937
Doctor Eugene H. Dibble, Jr.
Manager, Veterans Administration Facility
Tuskegee, Alabama
Dear Doctor Dibble:
   During the winter of 1937–1938 five years will have elapsed since the first clinical study was made of the individuals included in the untreated syphilis

6. The Tuskegee Veterans Hospital

project in Macon County. I am sure that you are thoroughly familiar with the details of this study and with the publication of results which was reported about a year ago in the Journal of the American Medical Association.

As you also know we are greatly interested in learning the ultimate fate of the individuals with untreated syphilis as well as the control individuals who presumably do not have syphilis. For the past two or three years a special attempt has been made to bring to necropsy study all of the individuals who have died. An opportunity second only in importance to necropsy study is periodic clinical observation.

If the agencies which are cooperating with the Public Health Service are interested we propose during the winter of 1937–1938 to assign an officer to Tuskegee whose duty it will be to examine clinically and do a thorough laboratory study on all of the individuals both syphilitic and nonsyphilitic included in this investigation. The purpose of this letter is to inquire whether the facilities in your institution will be placed at the disposal of our officer. If so, do you have between your hospital and the John A. Andrew Memorial Hospital all of the facilities which will be necessary to complete the cardiologic examination outlined on the accompanying form, with the exception of the electrocardiographic study?

Sincerely yours,
(Sgd) Thomas Parran
Surgeon General[39]

Dr. Dibble replied on February 12, advising Dr. Parran that he was referring the request to use the facilities at the Veterans Hospital and the John A. Andrew Memorial Hospital for the syphilis study, to the medical director of the Veterans Administration. The approval came just six days later.

February 18, 1937
Surgeon General
United States Public Health Services
Washington, D.C.

Dear Sir:

Your letter of February 9, 1937, addressed to the Manager of the Veterans Administration Facility, Tuskegee, Alabama, in which you request that that facility cooperate with you in the study which is being carried on in Macon County, Alabama, relative to Untreated Syphilis in the Male Negro has been referred to this office.

You are advised that I have this date authorized the Manager of the Tuskegee Facility to cooperate with your representative in completing this study.

Very truly yours,
(Sgnd) Frank T. Hines
Administrator[40]

The Tuskegee Veterans Hospital and Its Black Physicians

And so the Tuskegee VA Hospital, whose mission and purpose was to provide medical treatment and care for black veterans, became a partner in the Tuskegee Untreated Syphilis Study.

All of the Alabama men were brought to the modern Veterans Administration Hospital in Tuskegee and were examined by a public health service physician. Whenever diagnostic questions arose, consultation with specialists in ophthalmology, neurology, and cardiology was readily available and often utilized.[41]

In an interview, James T. Braye, former director of the hospital's human resource department and a nephew of Toussaint Tildon, stated that "many VA physicians were called in to work with patients from the syphilis study for surgery and treatment of special medical or psychiatric conditions. The treatment was usually not documented because they weren't supposed to treat non-VA patients. The facility was also used to perform autopsies on the study participants."[42]

There is evidence that at least two of Dr. Fuller's trainees participated in the study, although the extent of their participation is uncertain. In the outline for a proposal to continue the study dated November 1951, it is stated, "Dr. G. C. Branche, Chief of Clinical Services at V.A., has promised assistance from his medical residents."[43] As manager of the hospital, Dr. Toussaint Tildon's approval was requested for the use of a VA vehicle to transport study participants in a report by Dr. P. J. Pesare of the USPHS in 1948.

> I presume Dr. Hogan has informed you of my request via telephone for assistance in order to improve our transportation scheme to a more practical level. According to the plan which has been in operation—we are dependent on our nurse, Miss Rivers—to bring the patients to the Veteran's Hospital for examination. She has her private auto—a 5 passenger sedan. Not more than five appointments can be made daily since transportation facilities are limited to five persons. Should one or two of the patients receiving notification feel indisposed, frightened, or actually fail to receive their letters, that means that I don't see more than three to four patients on that day. I feel confident that as many as eight patients could be handled satisfactorily if this bottle-neck could be overcome.
>
> I have discussed the matter with Dr. Tildon, the superintendent of the Veteran's Hospital. He has been very cooperative and sympathetic. He is ready and willing to assign a Veterans Administration station wagon and driver to transport these patients to and from the hospital. All he needs is a clearance for such a cooperative service—from the Veterans Administration in Washington.

6. The Tuskegee Veterans Hospital

Apparently there are many questions asked when it comes to the justification for providing such transportation facilities. The penalties imposed for breach of regulations are quite severe.[44]

Reports were regularly given at monthly meetings of the Tuskegee Medical Society. While the purpose of these reports was to provide research updates, they often contained racial comments and stereotypes as seen in the following:

> Out of 2,107 persons who were given a blood test, regardless of whether they had or had not received previous treatment, from December 1939 to May 1, 1940, 451 of them were positive or about 20.4% of the 2,107 were positive. 273 were females, 150 males, or 36.0% were males and 63.4% were females. This figure for the females is the reverse of what is generally found, as most positives have been found in males in other places. I believe that the female is more promiscuous than the male, since the male gives little support for her keep and naturally she socks any aid possible and, as a bounty, she indulges in sex. Many of my patients have had children by 3 or 4 different men and even given each child the name of each father. If any group of people have more syphilis than any other group it is because of inadequate care, poverty, ignorance and lack of morals.[45]

Several years later, there appeared to be an attempt by the USPHS to redirect the study's funding for autopsies from the Tuskegee Institute to the Macon County Health Department.

> November 27, 1941
> Dr. R. A. Vonderlehr
> U. S. Public Health Service
> Washington, D. C.
> Dear Doctor Vonderlehr:
>
> When it comes time for you to renew the Milbank appropriation for taking care of autopsies in the untreated syphilis study, I wish that you would give some consideration to placing the Fund with Macon County Health Department instead of the Tuskegee Institute. The officials at Tuskegee Institute are not the same ones that you and I had such fine cooperation with a few years ago. They know nothing about the study, they do nothing for the patients, and for two years autopsies have been done in undertaker parlors. This proved to be more convenient for undertakers, and for us. The Institute will pay no bills that Dr. J. A. Kenney does not approve. Dr. Kenney knows nothing of what is going on, is always hard to find and is out of town a good deal of the time.
>
> If you will allow us to disburse the fees, it will give us a closer tie-in with the families and undertakers, whereas at present, they feel that Tuskegee Institute

The Tuskegee Veterans Hospital and Its Black Physicians

is giving them this help. They have lost sight of the fact the Health Department is still doing its part in keeping the study going along according to plans.

Please advise me of your reaction to this proposition. Its sole aim is to place the Health Department more in the 'spot light' than Tuskegee Institute.

Sincerely yours,
(Sgnd) Murray Smith, M.D.
Special Expert, V.D.
United States Public Health Service[46]

An attempt to downplay the involvement of the Tuskegee Institute in the 1972 federal investigation of the Untreated Syphilis Study is seen in correspondence between two members of the Ad Hoc Advisory Panel.

> I became convinced, during our field visit, that every possible precaution should be taken in any subsequent reports made by our Panel, including and especially our final report, to distinguish between the study that has gone on since 1932 under the auspices of the U.S. Public Health Service, and Tuskegee Institute, including the latter's hospital and clinics. Not only is it clear that Tuskegee Institute has done for many years, a great pioneering educational job in the deep South, along with its work in the medical and health fields. It is also clear that its present contributions, and realistic planning for the immediate future, are factors that our Panel appreciates, and that we ought, therefore, in a proper way, include such praiseworthy comments at some appropriate point in our reports. Such a position would include statements demonstrating that the connection between the whole Macon County syphilis project and Tuskegee Institute was at all times minimal, and that any negative criticism of aspects of that project that have been made or shall be made by our Panel will make it clear that Tuskegee Institute was and is not accountable for any such errors.[47]

Responding to the federal report of the investigation, the Tuskegee VA also attempted to minimize the facility's participation in the syphilis study. The hospital's director, Dr. Robert S. Wilson, denied that the hospital had any direct involvement, stating: "The Veterans' Administration would not condone or approve of such as this."[48]

The United States' increasing involvement in World War II created a new challenge to the syphilis study researchers. Some of the control cases who had developed syphilis were getting notices from the draft boards to be treated. When notified of the situation, Dr. R. A. Vsonderlehr, Assistant Surgeon General, Division of Venereal Diseases, UPHS, directed Dr. Murray Smith, USPHS health officer in Macon County, to "confer with the chairman of the local Selective Service

6. The Tuskegee Veterans Hospital

Board, who I know is Mr. J. F. Segrest. I believe he is an old friend of yours and I would inform him of all the circumstances connected with the study. It is entirely probable that if you place a list of the male Negroes included in this study in Mr. Segrest's hands, he will cooperate with you in the completion of the investigation. The present study of untreated syphilis is of great importance from a scientific standpoint. It represents one of the last opportunities which the science of medicine will have to conduct an investigation of this kind."[49]

In a letter dated August 6, 1942, from Dr. Smith to Dr. R. A. Vonderlehr, he reported, "So far, we are keeping the known positive patients from getting treatment.... Shall we withhold treatment from a control case who has developed syphilis?"[50]

Although penicillin was introduced in 1942 and acknowledged by the Public Health Service by the early 1950s as an effective treatment for late and latent syphilis, treatment continued to be withheld from the participants in the Tuskegee study.[51] It was the judgment of the Tuskegee Syphilis Study Ad Hoc Advisory Panel that serious ethical, legal, and scientific violations were made in the research project.

That penicillin therapy should have been made available to the participants in this study especially as of 1953 when penicillin became generally available. Withholding penicillin, after it became generally available, amplified the injustice to which this group of human beings had already been subjected. The scientific merits of the Tuskegee Study are vastly overshadowed by the violation of basic ethical principles pertaining to human dignity and human life imposed on the experimental subjects.[52]

The 1940s

By 1940, the town of Tuskegee had more than 1000 middle-class black professionals living and working in the community.[53] Between 1940 and 1950, the number of blacks occupying white-collar position increased by 172 percent and the number holding skilled jobs more than doubled.[54] Most of the new employment was provided by the VA hospital, its staff growing rapidly to accommodate the influx of disabled black veterans from the war.

The Tuskegee Veterans Hospital and Its Black Physicians

Macon County's population now had several options in the provision of medical care. The county's health department provided services to those who were unable to pay for care and for those suffering from syphilis and other venereal diseases. The department was staffed by one health officer and two venereal disease clinicians, one at full-time, the other part-time. Other health care providers included ten physicians in private practice, the John Andrew Memorial Hospital, which was a private hospital, and the veterans hospital for ex-servicemen. Four of the private physicians were located in Tuskegee, two were at the Tuskegee Institute, and the remaining four were in nearby towns. Eight were white and two were black.[55]

Between 1932 and 1942, the number of black physicians practicing in the South dropped from 2,295 to 2,018. Following the migration of Southern blacks to Northern cities, African American physicians were increasingly leaving the South, creating a void within the rural and poorest black populations in the Jim Crow states.[56] Kentucky, Tennessee, Alabama, and Mississippi experienced a dramatic decline in the number of black physicians from 626 to 538 (14 percent).

By June 30, 1940, the scope of the services provided by the Veterans Administration for the care and treatment of veterans had grown and there had been a steady increase in the number of hospital beds made available at its facilities throughout the country. There were now 60,000 beds, 35,000 of them designated for veterans with mental and nerve disabilities; 20,000 reserved for general medical and surgical cases; and more than 5000 set apart for tuberculosis patients.[57]

The bed capacity at the Tuskegee Veterans Hospital, No. 91, had also increased from 600 when it opened in 1923 to 1,558 following the remodeling of three wards. The number of beds available for neuropsychiatric patients was now 1,087 and there were 411 beds designated for general medical and surgical patients. The Tuberculosis Unit had been closed and those patients were transferred to the hospital in Oteen, North Carolina. A special ward at the Tuskegee facility housed patients who were diagnosed with both tuberculosis and neuropsychiatric disorders. Sixty-three buildings were now situated on fifty-five of the 486 acres that make up the hospital grounds. Approximately 110 acres were under cultivation, with the rest of the land dotted with trees and woodlands.

6. The Tuskegee Veterans Hospital

The number of hospital employees had also increased from the 176 who were on duty when the facility opened in 1923 to 645—38 physicians, 2 dentists, 77 nurses, 269 hospital attendants, and 93 dietetic employees, with the remainder consisting of administrative officials, technicians, clerical employees, and various types of custodial employees.[58]

Dr. Fuller's trainees had earned the respect of the Veterans Administration for their work at the Tuskegee facility and had assumed positions of authority. They were also beginning to gain professional recognition and accreditation. Toussaint Tildon had been promoted to the position of clinical director and manager of the hospital by General Omar Bradley upon the resignation of Dr. Dibble in 1946. Simon O. Johnson was now the chief of service and in 1947, was appointed to the American Board of Psychiatry and Neurology. In that same year,

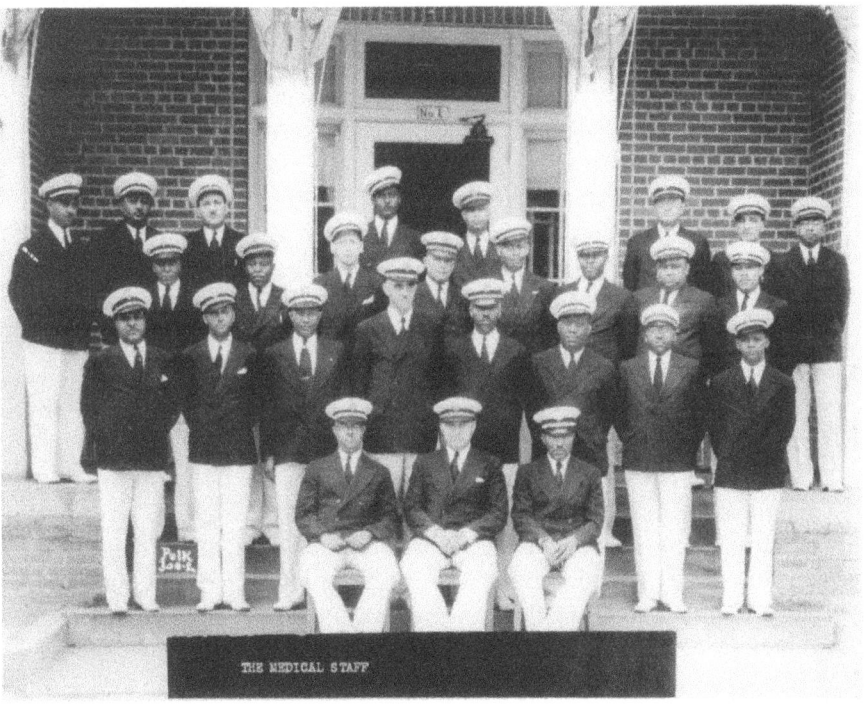

The medical staff, Tuskegee Veterans Hospital, 1944. Seated, left to right, Drs. Tildon, Dibble, and Branche; second row, far right, Dr. Davis; third row, far left, Dr. Johnson (Tuskegee University Archives, Tuskegee, Alabama).

The Tuskegee Veterans Hospital and Its Black Physicians

Harvey Davis was appointed to the American Board of Physical Medicine and Rehabilitation. George Branche had been promoted to chief of clinical services in 1946. He was appointed to the American Board of Psychiatry and Neurology that same year and in 1944 was the recipient of the E. S. Jones Award for Outstanding Research in Medical Science. On the local level, he served on the Committee for the Development of Psychopathic Hospitals and Other Mental Health Resources, sponsored by the Tuskegee Medical Society, where he led the study of local needs and the feasibility of starting a mental health program to include children, college students, and adults.

The facility was designated as a training center for physicians. Five physicians had completed the training by 1940, and, as a result, were promoted from the grade of junior physician to associate physician. The first cadet nurses program was inaugurated in 1944 and approximately 20 nurses from several schools were assigned to the Tuskegee VA for clinical training. In 1949, two American Medical Association-approved residency programs were established: one in internal medicine and surgery, and another in psychiatry. Residents were taught and supervised by medical school faculty from Emory University and the University of Alabama. The newsletter of the American Psychiatric Association stated on September 15, 1949, "In Tuskegee, Alabama, the all-colored staff and patients at the VA Hospital rank high in humanitarian efforts, given and received. A training program in Psychiatry is about to be started."[59]

The Veterans Administration's medical program came of age in 1946 with the creation of the Department of Medicine and Surgery by the 79th Congress. Public Law 293 permitted the inauguration of a program of graduate training in the VA in association with medical schools.[60] After being administered for twenty-five years under civil service, the now independent department was headed by a chief medical director.[61] The reason for the expansion of clinical facilities of the VA and educational facilities of medical institutions was to provide better care to veterans through cooperation in introducing graduate training programs in VA hospitals. A second objective was to recruit physicians for VA hospitals near medical schools. Tuskegee participated fully in these reorganizations and established associations with the University of Alabama and Emory medical schools.

6. The Tuskegee Veterans Hospital

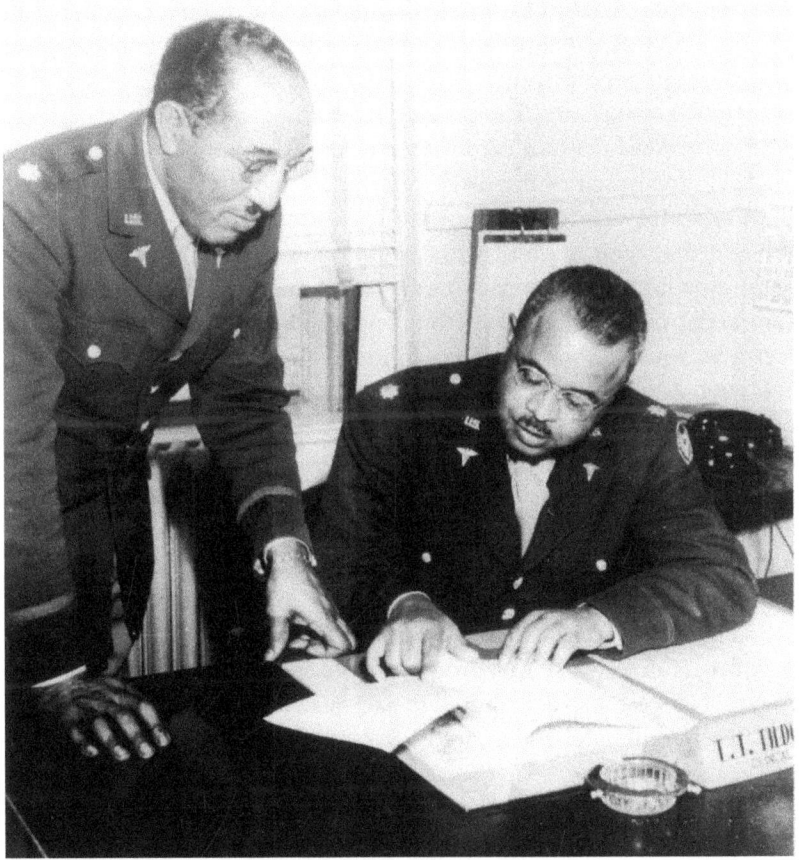

George Branche (standing) and Toussaint Tildon, February 1944 (Tuskegee University Archives, Tuskegee, Alabama).

The Tuskegee hospital remained a segregated hospital, admitting only black veterans. By this time, numbers of black veterans were also being treated in segregated wards in many of the Veterans Administration facilities throughout the country. Of the 127 VA hospitals, twenty-four had separate wards for black patients, but most of the nineteen VA hospitals in the South, with the exception of the Tuskegee VA, refused admission to blacks except in emergencies.[62] It was designated as an NP (general medical facility), and its patients consisted of two main types: neuropsychiatric and general medical.

The Tuskegee Veterans Hospital and Its Black Physicians

The neuropsychiatric cases were divided into functional disorders (60 percent), such as schizophrenia and manic depression, and neurological disorders (10 percent), such as various types of brain disease and diseases of the spinal cord. The majority of the medical cases were patients with cardiovascular and cardiorenal diseases.

The treatment of the black veteran was not unlike that provided for the white veteran, with some exceptions. For instance, it was thought that their immunity to certain types of parasitic diseases and disproportionate lack of resistance to others made it necessary that careful consideration be given to the use of viruses. Another important factor to consider was the low economic status of many of the black veterans. Because their average age was 45 and there were fewer job opportunities for them, it was important that they be fully rehabilitated before they were discharged to the community. It became the hospital's job not only to treat the disease or condition that was making the veteran ill but to also be responsible to rehabilitate him to the point where he would be able to make a successful adjustment when he returned to his home.

The library played an important role in the hospital's rehabilitation program. Books were not only available for those coming into the library, but were also distributed to patients on the wards. A press club, debate club, philatelic club, and book review club were just some of the groups for patients that were organized by the librarian. For blind patients, classes were offered in Braille which enabled them to read and in many cases to write.

Treatment for the hospital's large group of psychiatric patients consisted primarily of occupational and recreational therapies. Patients were assigned to the woodworking shop, paint shop, farm, landscape section and to the sewing room where bath hammocks and pajamas were made. The bath hammocks were used for the extended therapeutic baths for acutely disturbed patients; the pajamas were used by the patients; and the vegetables and hogs from the farm were utilized in the Dietary Department. Higher functioning patients were often assigned to the laundry, utilities, and dietetic departments as well as used as messengers.

For the lower functioning and regressed patients, there was an elementary-level training program that was based on a kindergarten

6. The Tuskegee Veterans Hospital

model. Patients were taught simple rules of conduct, to perform simple tasks, to coordinate their efforts, and proper hygiene. When these skills had been accomplished, they were taught basket weaving and rug making. For those patients who achieved success in these basic training levels, they could then move into more advanced outside occupational therapy projects and eventually be able to return to his home for a trial visit or discharge.

Recreational activities included seasonal games such as baseball, volley ball, croquet, and tennis as well as hiking, swimming, and dancing. Movies were provided twice weekly and radio programs played daily. Billiards, checkers, dominoes and card games were also available.

World War II

When the United States entered World War II in 1941, some blacks were already in the service and more were being drafted under the Selected Service Act, signed by President Franklin Roosevelt in 1940. But until the end of the war, most black servicemen were quartered in segregated units and were not utilized in battle. Secretary of War Henry Stimson said, "In the draft we are preparing to give the Negroes a fair shot in every service, even in aviation where I doubt very much they will not produce disaster there. Nevertheless, they are going to have a try but I hope for heavens sakes they don't mix the white and colored troops together in the same units for then we shall certainly have trouble."[63]

In 1920, the navy had adopted a policy of total exclusion of blacks, which was lifted in 1932 to allow them to enlist only as mess stewards. Protesting that they were "sea going bellhops, chambermaids and dishwashers" and that they had little chance for advancement in rank and received less pay than white sailors, a group of black sailors aboard the ship *Philadelphia* described their complaints in a letter to the *Pittsburgh Courier* in the summer of 1940. The men were immediately discharged as "undesirables," with a statement by the navy that enlisting "men of the colored race" for any branch of the naval service except as messmen was not in the best interest of a ship's efficiency.[64]

The Tuskegee Veterans Hospital and Its Black Physicians

The policy against enlisting men of color in the Marines was even more blunt, as indicated by the commandant of the Marines, Major General Thomas Holcomb: "If it were a question of having a Marine Corps of 5,000 whites or 250,000 Negroes, I would rather have the whites."[65]

As the United States mobilized for war, black physicians and leaders of the National Medical Association queried the War Department about their ability to serve their country. Remembering the segregation that they experienced during World War I, they wanted assurance that black physicians would be integrated into the medical corps and not be required to practice in separate facilities for sick and wounded black troops. Dr. G. Hamilton Francis stated: "Our nation is again preparing to defend itself against aggression from without. Today, we are ready and willing to contribute all of our skill and energy and to wholeheartedly enlist our services as members of the medical profession, but we must be permitted to take our right place, as evidenced by our training, experience, and ability.[66]

In a meeting with President Roosevelt in September 1940, Civil Rights leaders A. Philip Randolph and Walter White expressed their dismay over the racist policies in the military, stating that African Americans felt that they were not wanted in the armed forces of the country, even though they had fought in all wars since the American Revolution. The president replied that although there was a War Department pledge to recruit African Americans in all branches of the armed forces, including combat services, this policy was only in effect during a war. Despite the United States' entry into the war a few months later, the discrimination against the use of blacks in most branches of the service persisted.

The navy continued to bar blacks from serving on men-of-war because many officers thought that they did not have the skills and aptitude for sea duty. The Bureau of Naval Personnel believed that the African American's unfamiliarity with the sea "gave him a fear of water."[67] Randolph and White, having received no response from the president after their appeal regarding racial discrimination in the military, met with Eleanor Roosevelt. Ms. Roosevelt, an outspoken advocate for Civil Rights, urged the War Department to promise that black units would be formed in each branch of the military and would include aviation training. But the department refused to integrate the races.

6. The Tuskegee Veterans Hospital

"The policy of the War Department is not to intermingle colored and white enlisted personnel in the same regimental organizations. This policy has been proven satisfactory over a long period of years and to make changes would produce situations destructive to morale and detrimental to the preparation for national defense."[68] Despite the "Separate but Equal" policy touted by the War and Navy departments, black troops were given inferior services or were excluded from them entirely. Treatment was provided to sick and injured black soldiers in segregated wards in hospitals located on military bases and black physicians were allowed to treat only black military personnel.

The Tuskegee VA reached a peak bed capacity of approximately 2100 during World War II. When the United States entered the war in 1941, many of the younger hospital employees were called into the service and it was difficult to recruit adequate numbers of competent replacements. In response to the staffing crisis, Congress passed legislation to allow VA medical and dental personnel to be inducted into the service as medical officers. In February 1944, the hospital's medical and dental officers went on active duty with the U.S. army. The managers of all VA hospitals were given the rank of colonel and Dr. Dibble became the first U.S. black medical officer to be commissioned at this rank.[69]

As the war continued, the need for new recruits eventually forced the mobilization of large numbers of African Americans. Those black military regiments that were stationed in the United States were confronted with prejudice, not only in the South, but in other areas of the country as well as in territories such as Hawaii and Alaska. In Louisiana, a private, T. Nicklus, was pushed and hit by a train conductor. When he protested, the conductor shouted, "Give me the ticket, Nigger." A black soldier in Texas reported that the black troops were "not even as good as dogs, much less soldiers, even our General on the post hates the sight of a colored soldier ... and let me tell you it couldn't be any worse than hell itself."[70]

Tuskegee was home to the Tuskegee Army Flying School, the segregated unit for training black cadets in aviation instruction. In his 1940 presidential campaign, Franklin Roosevelt announced that the army would train blacks as aviators. This decision was in response to demands that black soldiers be treated more equitably in the new war effort than they had been during World War I.[71] The Tuskegee Institute,

The Tuskegee Veterans Hospital and Its Black Physicians

in its tradition of seeking new opportunities for blacks, lobbied to bring the aviation training program to Tuskegee. Although the school brought a boost to the area's economy because of the expenditures by the cadets and support troops, there was a great deal of hostility directed at them by the town's white citizens. The presence of 3000 young black men in uniform intensified the racial anxieties of the 1000 white Tuskegeeans. Many of the black soldiers were well-educated Northerners who were unaccustomed to the blatant prejudice of the small Alabama town. Recalling his experiences during his assignment at the flight school, a cadet stated: "It was a miserable place for [black] American servicemen to live and train to fight the enemies of the nation."[72]

The Tuskegee Airmen, an all-black pursuit squadron, was the only unit in the army to have black officers. Highly regarded and recognized for their heroism, they destroyed 409 enemy aircraft, sank an enemy destroyer, and knocked out many ground installations.[73]

With the increase in casualties among the white troops, it became necessary to replace them with blacks in combat situations. The 92nd Division was reactivated in 1942, but was faced with problems in training for combat duty. The test scores for the recruits were low, with none of the men placing in Class I, 10 percent in Class II, 56 percent in lower classifications, and 13 percent receiving no score because they were illiterate. Special classes were scheduled as well as extra training for those men who were not capable of fulfilling the basic training requirements.[74] Two of the 92nd Division's regiments, the 370th Regimental Combat Team (the old Buffalo Soldiers regiment) and the 371st Regiment, received many decorations and citations for their performance in combat. Their success and achievements of other black troops in World War II would later be used to support arguments for full integration.

Desegregation of the Veterans Administration

Efforts to desegregate veterans hospitals had begun shortly after World War II. In October 1945, representatives of Civil Rights groups

6. The Tuskegee Veterans Hospital

and black medical organizations met with General Paul R. Hawley, the medical director of the Veterans Administration, demanding the complete integration of the agency's hospitals.[75] Several years later, in 1948, the National Medical Association, following the desegregation of the armed forces by the president, asked the newly-appointed head of the Veterans Administration, General Omar Bradley, for a conference to plan for a similar desegregation of the VA.[76] General Bradley met with a group of black physicians and citizens and then requested that his medical director, General Hawley, hold meetings to hear both sides of the proposal. On the second day of a meeting in Washington, D.C., General Bradley announced that Truman was signing a presidential order to desegregate all VA hospitals.

The 1950s

The 1500 people who worked at the Tuskegee VA hospital by 1950 were an important force in the accelerated fight for voting rights. Beginning in the mid–1940s, efforts were made to challenge the rule that blacks wishing to register to vote in an election were required to bring vouchers affirming their right to vote. It was not unusual for the Board of Registrars to refuse to accept most black voters. The first objections to the board's procedures had been made by a small group of Tuskegee Institute professors and administrators, but soon, large numbers of VA and Tuskegee Army Air Field employees were joining the protest.

A suit was filed in the Alabama circuit court by twenty-five black voting applicants, charging that the board had unfairly denied them the right to vote.[77] Because, as federal employees, VA workers were immune to pressure from local whites, it was decided to file a similar, simultaneous suit in federal district court in Montgomery, with William P. Mitchell, a VA employee, as the plaintiff. Mitchell, had taken a job as an orderly at the hospital in 1935 and was soon trained to be a physical therapist, a position he would hold for thirty-five years. Aided by the local NAACP branch, which raised the money to pay for the litigation, the plaintiffs were represented by Arthur Shores, a Birmingham attorney who handled NAACP cases in Atlanta. Many of the applicants rejected were employed either at the hospital or the airfield. Another plaintiff and VA employee, Daniel L. Beasley, demonstrated the attitude and experience of those who were challenging the voter registration protocol for blacks: "When I came out of the army I was determined to register to vote.... I born here. I was a college graduate. I had been in the army.... I had never been in jail.... I just figured I ought to be registered."[78]

Citizen participation in public health planning in the state of Alabama rarely included the African American population. Neither public or professional channels were available to blacks. Typically, the method by which decisions were reached on health matters was through the contact of a black community leader with a health officer, a member of the county board of health, or in some cases, the probate judge or another county official. The person approached would then present the case at planning conferences or sessions. Black physicians continued to be excluded from membership in county and state medical societies, the American Medical Association, and the boards of health.

With the construction of a new clinical building in 1951, the hospital expanded its medical and surgical services and staff.[79] In that same year, Harvey Davis was promoted to the position of chief of physical medicine and rehabilitation services.

By the end of the 1950s, there had been a change in the hospital's administration. Dr. Prince P. Barker, who had served as chief of the neuropsychiatric service, and later as director of professional services, succeeded Dr. Tildon on February 1, 1958. Serving only two years, during which he revamped and upgraded the psychiatric services, Dr. Barker retired in 1959. He was succeeded by Dr. Howard W. Kenney, the son of Dr. John Kenney, the former director of the John A. Andrew Hospital at Tuskegee Institute.

Korean Conflict

Even though President Truman had issued his executive order for mandating desegregation of the military several years earlier, some all-black units were still in existence at the beginning of the Korean conflict. By 1951, a high rate of black enlistments (one out of every four new recruits in the army), combined with a shortage of men in white

6. The Tuskegee Veterans Hospital

units, forced the integration of both training and combat units.[80] Most white soldiers reported that they had few problems with the absorption of blacks into their units. Although racist comments were sometimes made and a fight would break out between the white and the black recruits, it was usually resolved by the parties involved.

Following the Korean conflict, the decision was made to retain the draft in order to create a "peacetime military" for deployment around the world. By 1956, the remnants of the Jim Crow military had vanished and men of all races and social class were required to serve their country for a minimum of two years.

7

1986

Thirty-Seven Years Later

The Tuskegee Veterans Hospital began as a neuropsychiatric and tuberculosis facility, with a small medical section. In the early days, the hospital's treatment model for psychiatric patients was custodial, authoritarian and disciplinary. This institutional model was the accepted means of treatment at a time when reactions of patients to repressive strictures of hospitalization were not yet understood. Over a period of time, there was a move toward a more humane emphatic regard for the mentally ill. Known as the "moral treatment of the insane," the movement was sparked by newspapers, magazines, and critics during the mid–1930s. With the introduction of insulin shock therapy in 1938, followed by electro-shock, psycho-surgery, and tranquilizers, many patients with mental illnesses that were previously untreatable, could now benefit from a variety of therapeutic measures.

Throughout the years, there were many well-known personalities who visited the Tuskegee VA. Two of the most distinguished were President Franklin D. Roosevelt on March 30, 1936, and Mrs. Eleanor Roosevelt, who visited the hospital for the first time on September 14, 1939, and again on March 27, 1941. Visits of inspection were made periodically by General Omar Bradley, Brigadier General B. O. Davis, Sr., and his son, Colonel B. O. Davis, Jr.[1] During World War II, stars of stage and screen fame also came to the hospital to visit with the sick and injured troops.

Racism continued to plague the Southern medical community into the 1960s. In 1953, the Medical Association of the State of Alabama

7. 1986

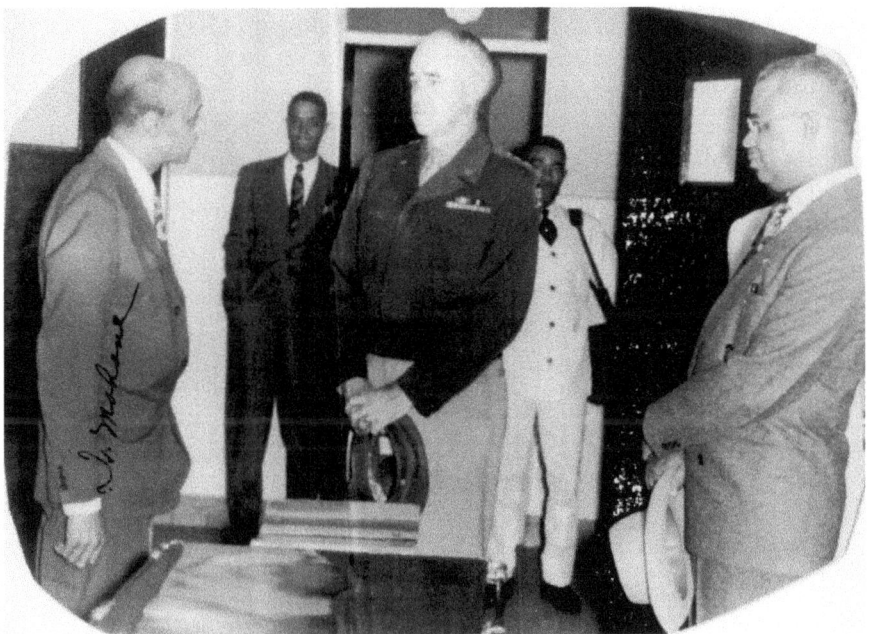

General Omar Bradley's visit to the Tuskegee Veterans Hospital, date unknown. With, left to right, Drs. Mahone, Branche and Tildon (Tuskegee University Archives, Tuskegee, Alabama).

directed its affiliates to admit black physicians. By 1965, despite continuing progress in the integration of medical associations, only four of Alabama's seventy local medical associations had granted membership to black physicians.[2]

Two major events led to the integration of hospitals in the South. With the passage of the Civil Rights Act of 1964, came sanctions imposed by the federal government for those hospitals that were not in compliance with the regulations for integration established by the legislation. A year later, the passage of Medicare provided financial support to hospitals for the medical treatment of elderly patients. In order to qualify for Medicare funding, hospitals were required to be in compliance with Title VI of the Civil Rights Act, which forbid the federal government from allocating funds to facilities that discriminated on the basis of race, creed, or national origin.[3]

The transformation of the Tuskegee VA hospital involved the

racial integration of patients and staff. Although originally established as a segregated facility, specifically for black veterans, full integration evolved without incident.[4] By 1960, the trend toward desegregation of the Tuskegee hospital was in evidence. A large number of white veterans had voluntarily joined the predominately black patient population. Two white nurses had served for a time on the medical services. One male white nursing assistant had been employed and others were applying. Harvey Davis' position as chief of physical medicine and rehabilitation was now held by a white physician.[5] With the desegregation of medical staff by the Veterans Administration outside the South, came the opening of opportunities that were previously closed to black physicians.

Almost all the hospital's pioneers had retired or passed on.

Simon O. Johnson

Simon O. Johnson was the first of Dr. Fuller's trainees to leave the Tuskegee VA. He accepted the position of Superintendent of the Lakin State Hospital in West Virginia in 1951. The hospital, which opened in 1926 as the State Hospital for Colored Insane, had an all-black staff and was only the second hospital in the United States to have a black administrator. It was located in predominately white Mason County, where it was assumed that any African American walking down the road was an escaped patient. All staff was housed at the facility, since they were unable to find housing in the area due to the hospital's distance from town (nine miles), a lack of transportation services, and segregated housing. A separate house for the superintendent was located across from the facility.[6]

The hospital gained a reputation as the "lobotomy capital of the East," when it became part of Dr. Walter Freeman's West Virginia Lobotomy Project. Dr. Freeman, a pioneer in lobotomy, offered to use the facility to perform lobotomies to bring in money for the hospital which the state had threatened to close. Johnson opened a medical center at the hospital in 1953, which attracted predominately white, private pay patients who were drawn to the facility by the positive reputation of the superintendent.

7. 1986

Dr. Johnson had a successful career in mental health administration, receiving the American Psychiatric Association Mental Health Achievement Award for his essay "The Making of a Hospital—New Concepts and New Personalities" and completed a certificate in Mental Hospital Administration from the American Psychiatric Association in 1955. He chaired the neuropsychiatry section of the National Medical Association from 1953 to 1959.

In 1958, he was elected president of the newly-integrated Mason County chapter of the American Medical Association in West Virginia. In later years, he held positions as the director of the Child Guidance Clinic at Memorial Hospital in West Virginia, on the staff of Holzer Hospital in Gallipolis, Ohio, and as a consultant to the Veterans Administration Regional Office in Huntington, West Virginia. He retired and moved to Detroit, Michigan, where he died on February 20, 1972, at age 77, following a brief illness.[7]

George Clayton Branche

Dr. Branche served continuously at the Tuskegee VA until his death, which came while working at the facility on July 2, 1956. In his thirty-three years of service, he had achieved much success and national recognition in the field of neuropsychiatry. Among his outstanding achievements was his contribution to research in the use of therapeutic quartan malaria in the treatment of neurosyphilis among African Americans. He was a fellow of the American Psychiatric Association, the National Medical Association, a member of the American Association for the Advancement of Sciences and the Association of Military Surgeons of the United States, and a diplomat of the American Board of Psychiatry and Neurology. He also served his country as a lieutenant colonel in the U.S. army during World War II.

Harvey Franklin Davis

Dr. Davis retired from the Tuskegee VA in 1955 and moved to Annapolis, Maryland, where he lived until the 1980s. He died in Mount

Vernon, New York, on January 29, 1986, at the age of 92. He is buried at the Baltimore National Cemetery.

Toussaint Tildon

The last of Dr. Fuller's trainees to leave the Tuskegee VA, Dr. Tildon retired on January 31, 1958, after thirty-four years of service, following an illness. During his career at the VA, he was known for being a mentor to black physicians as well as for his contributions to medicine. He conducted research on encephalitis in African American veterans and on syphilis and heart disease in patients with tuberculosis, publishing numerous articles on these topics. As the hospital's manager and director, he set high standards and achieved professional recognition for the hospital by securing accreditation for residency programs. He was a member of the Association of Military Surgeons and the American Heart Association, and a fellow of the National Medical Association, the American Medical Association, the American Psychiatric Association, and the John A. Andrew Clinical Society. He served his country in World War II, first as a lieutenant colonel and later as a colonel in the United States Medical Corps.

Toussaint Tildon died in Tuskegee on July 22, 1964, at the age of 71.

Solomon Carter Fuller

After 34 years of teaching and research, Dr. Fuller made the decision to retire from Boston University School of Medicine in 1933 when a white assistant professor was promoted to full professor and appointed head of the Neurology Department. During his last five years at the university, Fuller had served as the head of the department, but was never officially given the title. Despite his many achievements in medical science, the university never promoted him beyond the rank of associate professor. Rather than contesting the appointment, Fuller chose to leave. "I thoroughly dislike publicity of that sort and despise sympathy. I regard life as a battle in which we win or lose. As far as I am concerned, to be vanquished, if not ingloriously is not so bad after all. With the sort of work that I have done, I might have gone farther and reached a higher plan had it not been for my color."[8]

Fuller continued to work as a consultant at Westborough State Hospital and Framingham's Marlboro Hospital as well as the Pennsylvania State Hospital in Allentown until 1939 when his eyesight began to fail. Despite his blindness, he continued to practice psychiatry in Framingham with the assistance of a former student, Dr. Charles Pinderhughes. "He was slow, deliberate, thoughtful, persistent, considerate, but tough-minded. I would give the patient his physical examination and Dr. Fuller, blind and aged, would do the rest."[9]

Solomon Carter Fuller died on January 16, 1953, at the age of 80, following a long battle with diabetes and gastrointestinal cancer. The recognition of Dr. Fuller's accomplishments did not come until many years later, when, in 1972, the American Psychiatric Association recognized him as the first black psychiatrist in the United States and one of the "great men of American psychiatry."[10] In 1976, the Dr. Solomon Carter Fuller Mental Health Center was built through the collaborative efforts of the local, state, and national associations for mental health, Boston University Division of Psychiatry, and local community organizations. The building, located adjacent to Boston University Medical Center, was designed to provide facilities for psychiatric outpatient services, community education, and research.

Of the many affirmations of Dr. Fuller's important contributions to medicine, there was one that he received and especially treasured in his later years. It was a letter sent to him in 1950 by Dr. Eugene Dibble, secretary-treasurer of the John A. Andrew Clinical Society.

> We shall always remember the very fine part that you had in training there in Boston the original group of psychiatrists that came to start the Veterans Hospital in Tuskegee. Of that original group, Tildon, Branche, and Davis are still here, Tildon and Branche occupying the two highest positions in the hospital, Davis heading the Department of Physical Medicine and the only Diplomate of the American Board of Physical Medicine that we have in our group. The other member, S. C. Johnson, is now head of the State Institution at Lakin, West Virginia.
> He too, is a Diplmate of the American Board. It certainly must make you feel very proud to know that you had a great deal to do with training of these young men who have done so much in the field in which you started them off.[11]
> We can assure you that in opening the psychiatric meeting this year, you will be given due credit for the tremendously fine part that you played in the

starting and the development of this great work so closely allied and associated with the work of Dr. Washington, the founder of Tuskegee Institute.

Fuller and His Trainees: The Legacy of Tuskegee

For many years, the town of Tuskegee has lived with the stigma of the Tuskegee Syphilis Study and the myths surrounding it. The study was terminated in 1972. In 1974, the National Research Act was signed into law, creating the National Commission for the Protection of Human Subjects of Biomedical and Behavioral Research and the federal government agreed to pay a settlement to the survivors and families of the participants.[12]

The study has often been cited as the cause of distrust of the medical system by blacks, often referred to as the "Tuskegee effect." This distrust has been blamed for undermining outreach efforts of health care providers, including childhood immunizations, flu vaccinations and AIDS education programs.

But there is another legacy of Tuskegee—one that is an important addition to the history of Alabama, the history of medicine, and to African American history. It is the story of four doctors, who, inspired and trained by America's first black psychiatrist, went on to lead the black staff of the country's first hospital built to care for black veterans. With the eyes of the nation and the medical profession on the Tuskegee Veterans Hospital, professional recognition for black physicians in the hospital as well as at other government hospitals and medical facilities was achieved. In 1932, Peter Marshall Murray, president of the National Medical Association, called the hospital "a brilliant chapter in the annuals of Negro medicine ... [that] has also provided extraordinarily well for thousands of veterans of our race and given an opportunity to Negro professionals to demonstrate their fitness for this work."[13]

The contributions made by Solomon Carter Fuller, George C. Branche, Solomon O. Johnson, Harvey F. Davis, and Toussaint Tildon to improve the care for black veterans, in the promotion of blacks in the practice of medicine, through their research, and to the community at large will be a lasting legacy of their call to serve.

Chapter Notes

Introduction

1. Frederick Douglass, *Life and Times of Frederick Douglass*, reprinted from the revised edition of 1872 (New York: Collier Books, 1962), 337–338.
2. Bernard C. Nalty, *Strength for the Fights: A History of Black Americans in the Military* (New York: Free Press, 1986), 2.
3. Sidney Kaplan and Emma Nogrady Kaplan, *The Black Presence in the Era of the American Revolution* (Amherst: University of Massachusetts Press, 1989), 64–69.
4. *Lord Dunmore's Proclamation*, Digital History, retrieved August 6, 2005, from http://digitalhistory.uh.edu/learning history/revolution/dunsmore.com.
5. *Militia Act of 1792*, United States Statues at Large, Vol. 1, United States Congress, Public Acts of the Second Congress, First Session, Chapter 33.
6. James Roberts, *The Narrative of James Roberts, a Soldier Under General Washington in the Revolutionary War, and Under General Jackson at the Battle of New Orleans in the War of 1812: A Battle Which Cost Me a Limb, Some Blood and Almost My Life*, VIII (Chicago: Printed for the author, 1858), 18.
7. Peter M. Bergman, "The Negro Who Rode with Fremont in 1847," *Negro History Bulletin* 28, no. 2, 31–32.
8. Dudley T. Cornish, *The Sable Arm: Negro Troops in the Union Army, 1861–1865* (New York: Norton, 1965), 130.
9. David J. Eicher, *The Longest Night: A Military History of the Civil War* (New York: Simon & Schuster, 2001), 657.
10. *Official Records of the Union and Confederate Armies*, Series IV, Vol. III (Washington, D.C.: Government Printing Office, 1900), 1012–1013.
11. William E. Alt and Betty L. Alt, *Black Soldiers, White Wars* (Westport, CT: Praeger, 2002), 46.
12. Douglass, *Life and Times of Frederick Douglass*, 348.
13. Ibid., 354.
14. H. Roy Kaplan, *The Myth of Post-Racial America* (Lanham, MD: Rowman & Littlefield, 2011), 173.
15. Elsie Freeman, Wynell Burroughs Schamel, and Jean West, "The Fight for Equal Rights: A Recruiting Poster for Black Soldiers in the Civil War," *Social Education* 56 no. 2 (February 1992): 118–120.
16. Mark Grimsley, "Confederate Rage, Yankee Wrath—No Quarter in the Civil War," *Civil War History* 55, no. 3 (2009): 414–415.
17. Alt and Alt, *Black Soldiers, White Wars*, 52–53.
18. William Leckie, "The Buffalo Soldiers: A Narrative of the New Cavalry in the West," in *The Black Soldier from the Revolution to Vietnam*, Jay David and Elaine Crane, eds. (New York: William Morrow, 1971), 92.
19. Andrew D. Amron, "Reinforcing Manliness: Black State Militias, the Spanish-American War, and the Image of the African American Soldier, 1891–1900," *The Journal of African American*

Chapter Notes—1

History 97, no. 4 (Fall 2012): 404–405.

20. Harry E. Groves, "Separate but Equal—The Doctrine of Plessy v Ferguson," *Phylon* 12, no. 1 (1951): 66–72.

21. Amron, "Reinforcing Manliness," 410–411; William B. Gatewood, "Alabama's Negro Soldier Experiment, 1898–1899," *Journal of Negro History* 57 (October 1972): 339–343.

22. Alt and Alt, *Black Soldiers, White Wars*, 62.

23. Scott Brown, "White Backlash and the Aftermath of Fagen's Rebellion: The Fates of Three African American Soldiers in the Philippines, 1901–1902," *Contributions in Black Studies* 13 (1995): 165.

24. Gama L. Christian, "Brownsville Raid of 1906," *The Handbook of Texas Online*, Texas State Historical Association, retrieved July 22, 2012.

25. "The Brownsville Affair," *Dictionary of American History*, 2003, encylopedia.com, retrieved May 10, 2014.

26. Nalty, *Strength for the Fights*, 105.

27. Keith Krawczynski in *A Historic Context for the African American Military Experience*, eds. Steven D. Smith and James A. Zeidler (Champaign: United States Army Construction Engineering Research Laboratories, July 1998), 168.

28. "A French Directive," *The Crisis*, XVIII, May 1919, 16–18.

29. W. E. B. DuBois, *Ibid.*, 1–6.

30. Nalty, *Strength for the Fights*, 104–105.

31. Krawczynski, *A Historic Context for the African American Military Experience*, 155.

32. Nalty, *Strength for the Fights*, 109.

33. Jessie D. Ames in *Robert Russa Moton of Hampton and Tuskegee*, eds. William H. Hughes and Frederick D. Patterson (Chapel Hill: University of North Carolina Press, 1956), 153.

34. Krawczynski, *A Historic Context for the African American Military Experience*, 162.

35. W. E. B. DuBoi, in *Let Nobody Turn Us Around: Voices of Resistance, Reform, and Renewal, An African American Anthology*, eds. Manning Marable and Leith Mullins (Lanham, MD: Rowman & Littlefield, 2000), 242–243.

36. NAACP Papers, *Discrimination in the U.S. Armed Forces, 1918–1955*, Veterans Affairs Committee, Part 9, Series C, 10.

37. Krawczynski. *A Historic Context for the African American Military Experience*, 181.

Chapter 1

1. Vannessa N. Gamble, *Making a Place for Ourselves: The Black Hospital Movement, 1920–1945* (New York: Oxford University Press, 1995), 71.

2. Raymond Wolters, *The New Negro on Campus: Black College Rebellions of the 1920s* (Princeton: Princeton University Press, 1976), 151.

3. Editorial in *The Southern Workman* 52 (1923): 365.

4. Report of the Consultants on Hospitalization, November 16, 1921, Tuskegee Collection, National Library of Medicine, Washington, D.C., 53–54.

5. Albion L. Holsey, "A Man of Courage," in *Robert Russa Moton of Hampton and Tuskegee*, eds. William H. Hughes and Frederick D. Patterson (Chapel Hill: University of North Carolina Press, 1956), 128.

6. W. E. B. DuBois, "Opinion: The Tuskegee Hospital," *Crisis* 26 (July 1923): 106–107.

7. Letter from Walter White to Marianna G. Brubaker, July 16, 1923, Library of Congress NAACP Papers: Group I, Series C410, Container 410.

8. Gamble, *Making a Place for Ourselves*, 78.

9. Thomas Ward, *Black Physicians in the Jim Crow South* (Fayetteville: University of Arkansas Press, 2003), 250.

10. Robert Norrell, *Reaping the Whirlwind: The Civil Rights Movement in Tuskegee* (New York: Knopf, 1985), 26, 27.

11. Report of the Consultants on Hospitalization, letter of transmittal

Chapter Notes—1

submitted by William Charles White, Chairman, Frank Billings, John G. Bowman and George H. Kirby, Consultants on Hospitalization, dated February 28, 1923. Record Group 121, Records of the Public Building Service, Records of Consultants on Hospitalization, National Archives, Washington, D.C.

12. Frederick Douglass, *Life and Times of Frederick Douglass*, reprinted from the revised edition of 1872 (New York: Collier Books, 1962), 14.

13. Leon Litwack, "The Order of Black Freedom," in *The Southern Enigma: Essays on Race, Class and Folk Culture*, eds. Walter J. Fraser and Winfred B. Moore (Westport, CT: Greenwood Press, 1983), 19–20.

14. Wolters, *The New Negro on Campus: Black College Rebellions of the 1920s*, 156. Alan W. Ryff, *The Tuskegee Hospital Controversy, 1921–1924*, M. A. Thesis, University of Deleware, 1970.

15. "Hospital for Ex-servicemen to Be at Tuskegee," *Journal of the National Medical Association* 14 (1922): 208.

16. Wolters, *The New Negro on Campus*, 157.

17. U. S. Veterans Bureau field letter, February 3, 1923, NAACP Papers.

18. W. E. B. DuBois, "Opinion: The Tuskegee Hospital," *Crisis* 26 (July 1923): 107.

19. *The Tuskegee Student* 33, nos. 5–6 (March 1–15, 1923): 1–2.

20. "Negro Veterans' Hospital," *The Southern Workmen* 53 (July 1926): 106.

21. Albion L. Holsey, "The Negro Veterans' Hospital," *The Southern Workmen* 53 (July 1926): 305–314.

22. Wolters, *The New Negro on Campus*, 158.

23. "The Negro Veterans Hospital at Tuskegee," memorandum for the files, December 31, 1923, NAACP Papers.

24. Fourteenth Annual Report of the NAACP, 1923, p. 29, NAACP Papers.

25. Letter to Benjamin J. Davis from Albion Holsey, May 30, 1923, NAACP Papers.

26. Letter to Robert Moton, President, Tuskegee Institute from Robert Stanley, Medical Officer in Charge, U.S. Veterans Bureau, February 24, 1923, Robert Moton Papers, Box 95, File: Government Hospital 700, National Archives, Washington, D.C.

27. "The Tuskegee Hospital Muddle," *The Crisis* 28 (September 1923): 216.

28. George Christian, Notes on hospital situation, February 23, 1923, NAACP Papers.

29. Clifton O. Dummett and Eugene H. Dibble, "Historical Notes on the Tuskegee Veterans Hospital," *Journal of the National Medical Association* LIV, no. 52 (March 1962): 134.

30. Gamble, *Making a Place for Ourselves*, 84–86.

31. Albion L. Holsey letter to John Calhoun, July 6, 1923, Robert Moton Papers, Box 71, File: Government Hospital 700, National Archives, Washington, D.C.

32. Holsey letter to Calhoun.

33. Gamble, *Making a Place for Ourselves*, 6.

34. Holsey, "A Man of Courage," 132.

35. *Ibid.*, 133.

36. Editorial, *The Atlanta Independent*, May 24, 1923.

37. DuBois, "Opinion: Tuskegee Hospital," 107.

38. Wolters, *The New Negro on Campus*, 167.

39. Pete Daniel, "Black Power in the 1920s: The Case of the Tuskegee Veterans' Hospital," *Journal of Southern History* 36, no. 3 (August 1970): 372.

40. Albion L. Holsey, "The Negro Veterans' Hospital," *The Southern Workman* 55 (July 1926): 307.

41. John A. Kenney, "A Shortage of Negro Doctors: With Special Reference to Residents and Interns," *Annual Bulletin*, John A. Andrew Clinic, Tuskegee Institute, Alabama, 1940, 85.

42. Daniel, "Black Power in the 1920s," 374.

43. *New York Age*, July 1923.

44. Holsey, "A Man of Courage," 135.

45. *The Montgomery Advertiser*, July 4, 1923; *The Savannah Tribune*, July 4, 1923; Daniel, "Black Power in the 1920s,"

378–379; Ryff, *The Tuskegee Hospital Controversy, 1921–1924*, 26–27; "The Tuskegee Hospital Muddle," 217.

46. NAACP press release, July 10, 1923, Moton Papers, Box 125, File 941, University Archives, Tuskegee University, Tuskegee, Alabama.

47. "The Tuskegee Hospital muddle," 217.

48. *Ibid.*

49. Walter White in letter to J. Edgar Hoover, July 9, 1923, NAACP Papers.

50. Wolters, *The New Negro on Campus*, 173.

51. W. W. Campbell telegram to Robert R. Moton, July 4, 1923, Robert Moton Papers, Box 71, File: Government Hospital 700, National Archives, Washington, D.C.

52. W. E. B. DuBois, "No Compromise," *The Crisis* 72 (November 1923): 7–8.

53. Melvin Chisum letter to Hines, July 7, 1923, Director's Correspondence, NAACP Papers.

54. Fourteenth Annual Report of the NAACP, 1923, NAACP Papers.

55. Albion L. Holsey letter to James Weldon Johnson, April 2, 1923, Robert Moton Papers, Box 95, Tuskegee Archives; Gamble, *Making a Place for Ourselves*, 87.

56. *The Mobile Register*, July 5, 1923.

57. *Jackson Daily News*, quoted in *The New Age*, July 21, 1923.

58. *Norfolk Virginia-Pilot*, quoted in *Norfolk Journal and Guide*, July 21, 1923.

59. Gamble, *Making a Place for Ourselves*, 95.

60. "Kelly Miller Says," *Baltimore Afro-American*, August 31, 1923.

61. *Baltimore Afro-American*, September 7, 1923.

62. Robert Sharpley, ed., *Psychoanalysis, Psychotherapy, and the New England Medical Scene, 1844–1944* (New York: Science History Publishers, 1978), 192.

63. Mary Kaplan, *Solomon Carter Fuller: Where My Caravan Has Rested* (Lanham, MD: University Press of America, 2005), 65.

64. Gamble, *Making a Place for Ourselves*, 66, 100.

Chapter 2

1. Barbara McClure, "Medical Care Programs of the Veterans Administration," Congressional Research Service, Report No. 83–99 (Washington, D.C.: Library of Congress, May 1983), 1–4.

2. "VA History in Brief," Department of Veterans Affairs, 3–8, www.va.gov.cpa/publications/archives/docs/history, retrieved May 12, 2014.

3. William E. Alt and Betty L. Alt, *Black Soldiers, White Wars* (Westport, CT: Praeger, 2002), 41.

4. Alexander Thomas Augusta, *Journal of the National Medical Association* 44, no. 4 (July 1953): 328.

5. *Ibid.*, 327.

6. Jeanne Spurlock, *Black Psychiatrists and American Psychiatry* (Washington, D.C.: The American Psychiatric Association, 1999), 95–96.

7. "VA History in Brief," 7.

8. George F. Cannon, "The Negro Medical Profession and the United States Army," *Journal of the National Medical Association* 11, no. 1 (January–March 1919): 21–28.

9. Mary Kaplan, *Solomon Carter Fuller: Where My Caravan Has Rested* (Lanham, MD: University Press of America, 2005), 61–62.

10. Cannon, "The Negro Medical Profession and the United States Army," 21.

11. *Ibid.*, 24.

12. Louis T. Wright, "The New Doctor and the War," *Journal of the National Medical Association* 11, no. 4, 195–196.

13. Vanessa N. Gamble, *Making a Place for Ourselves: The Black Hospital Movement, 1920–1945* (New York: Oxford University Press, 1995), 6.

14. "History of the National Home for Disabled Volunteer Soldiers," National Park Service, U.S. Department of the Interior, www.nps.gov, retrieved May 16, 2014.

15. Judith G. Cetina, *A History of Veterans Homes in the United States, 1811–1930*, Ph.D. dissertation, Case Western Reserve University, Cleveland, Ohio, 1977, 30–39.
16. Martin Summers, "Suitable Care of the African When Afflicted with Insanity: Race, Madness, and Social Order in Comparative Perspective," *Bulletin of the History of Medicine* 84, no. 1 (Spring, 2010): 66–67; Gerald Grob, "Class, Ethnicity and Race in American Mental Hospitals," *Journal of the History of Medicine* 28 (1973): 207–229; Todd Savitt, *Medicine and Slavery* (Urbana: University of Illinois Press, 1981), 258–279; Peter McCandless, *Moonlight, Magnolias and Madness: Insanity in South Carolina from the Colonial Period to the Progressive Era* (Chapel Hill: University of North Carolina, 1996),75–77; Charles Pruhomme and David F. Musto, "Historical Perspectives on Mental Health and Racism," in *Racism and Mental Health*, eds. Charles Vert Willie, Bernard Kramer and Bertram Brown (Pittsburgh: University of Pittsburgh Press, 1973), 27–28.
17. Summers, "Suitable Care of the African when Afflicted with Insanity," 74.
18. Leland V. Bell, *Treating the Mentally Ill* (Westport, CT: Praeger, 1980), 59.
19. S. M. Buchanan, "Insanity in the Colored Race," *New York Medical Journal* 44 (1886): 69.
20. James H. Jones, *Bad Blood: The Tuskegee Syphilis Experiment* (New York: Free Press, 1981), 24–29.
21. Mary O'Malley, "Psychoses in the Colored Race," *American Journal of Insanity* 73 (1917): 326–327.
22. E. M. Green, "Manic-Depressive Psychoses in the Negro," *American Journal of Insanity* 73 (1917): 619–626.
23. Summers, "Suitable Care of the African When Afflicted with Insanity," 62.
24. *Ibid.*, 81.
25. Henry M. Hurd, William F. Drewry, Richard Dewey, Charles W. Pilgram, G. Alden Blumer, and T. J. W. Burgess, *The Institutional Care of the Insane in the United States and Canada*, Vol. I (Baltimore: Johns Hopkins University Press, 1916), 377–378.
26. Edward A. Strecker, "Military Psychiatry: World War I, 1917–1918," in *One Hundred Years of American Psychiatry* (New York: American Psychiatric Association, Columbia University Press, 1944), 77.
27. Albert Deutsch, *The Mentally Ill in America* (New York: Doubleday, 1938), 317–318.
28. Strecker, "Military Psychiatry," 403.
29. Caroline Alexander, "The Shock of War," *Smithsonian Magazine* 41, no. 5 (September 2010): 58–66.
30. Strecker, "Military Psychiatry," 412.
31. James H. Carter, "Alcoholism in Black Vietnam Veterans: Symptoms of Post-Traumatic Stress Disorder," *Journal of the National Medical Association* 74, no. 7 (1983): 655.
32. Strecker, "Military Psychiatry," 407.

Chapter 3

1. David Barton Smith, *Health Care Divided: Race and Healing a Nation* (Ann Arbor: University of Michigan Press, 1999), 14.
2. Vanessa N. Gamble, *Making a Place for Ourselves: The Black Hospital Movement, 1920–1945* (New York: Oxford University Press, 1995), 36.
3. Abraham Flexner and Henry Pritchett, *Medical Education in the United States and Canada* (New York: Carnegie Foundation for the Advancement of Teaching, Bulletin 4, 1910), 180.
4. Gamble, 19–20, 42.
5. *Ibid.*, 11.
6. Thomas Ward, Jr., *Black Physicians in the Jim Crow South* (Fayetteville: University of Arkansas Press, 2003), 50.
7. W. Montague Cobb, Reprint of Chapter X in *Negroes and Medicine*, eds.

C. Dietrict and C. Retzes (Cambridge: The Commonwealth Fund, Harvard University Press, 1958), 190–230.

8. Mary Kaplan, *Solomon Carter Fuller: Where my Caravan Has Rested* (Lanham, MD: University Press of America, 2005), 15–19.

9. *Ibid.*, 18.

10. Solomon Carter Fuller, "Anatomical Findings of General Paresis and Multiple Sclerosis in the Same Case," date unknown, Boston, Fuller Collection, Box 1, Francis A. Countway Library of Medicine.

11. Caroline Alexander, "The Shock of War," *Smithsonian* 41, no. 5 (September 2010), 59–60.

12. Kaplan, 74.

13. *Ibid.*, 25.

14. Lloyd Vernon Briggs, ed., *A History of the Psychopathic Hospital* (Boston: Wright and Potter Printing Company, 1922), 98.

15. Kaplan, 18.

16. Leland V. Bell, *Treating the Mentally Ill* (Westport, CT: Praeger, 1980), 87.

17. Briggs, 119.

18. "Preparing to Care for Shell-Shocked Men," *New York Times*, June 16, 1918.

19. Myrtelle M. Canavan, "Survey of the Work of the Director of the Psychopathic Hospital," in *A History of the Psychopathic Hospital*, ed. Lloyd V. Briggs, 193.

20. Kaplan, 65.

Chapter 4

1. Interview with Martie Elizabeth Branche Bauduit by Kelly Hughes, recorded on November 16, 2001, Maria Rogers Oral History Program, Carnegie Library.

2. Raymond Wolters, *The New Negro on Campus: Black College Rebellions of the 1920s* (Princeton: Princeton University Press, 1976), 278–293.

3. Interview with George C. Branche, III, September 20, 2013.

4. *Ibid.*

5. Boston University School of Medicine Alumni Medical Library, June 2014.

6. *Journal of the National Medical Association* 65, no. 1 (January 1973): 86.

7. Samuel L. Younge, *Journal of the National Medical Association* 56, no. 6 (1965): 565–566.

8. Nora Nercessian, *Against All Odds: The Legacy of Students of African Descent at Harvard Medical School Before Affirmative Action, 1850–1968* (Boston: Puritan Press, 2004), 39–40.

9. *New York Herald*, June 16, 1918.

Chapter 5

1. William Chafe, Raymond Gavins, and Robert Korstad, Eds., *Remembering Jim Crow* (New York: The New Press, 2001), 37.

2. *Ibid.*, 268.

3. Frederick Douglass, *Life and Times of Frederick Douglass*, reprinted from the revised edition of 1872 (New York: Collier Books, 1962), 397–399.

4. Leon F. Litwack, *Trouble in Mind: Black Southerners in the Age of Jim Crow* (New York: Alfred A. Knopf, 1998), 159.

5. "Negro Doctors and Hospitals," *Opportunity* 3 (1925): 227. John Kenney, "A Shortage of Negro Doctors: With Special Reference to Residents and Interns," *Annual Bulletin*, John A. Andrew Clinic, Tuskegee Institute, 1940, 85.

6. Edward Beardsley, "Dedicated Servants or Errant Professionals: The Southern Negro Physician Before World War II," in *The Southern Enigma: Essays on Race, Class, and Folk Culture*, eds. Walter Frasier, Jr., and Winfred B. Moore, Jr. (Westport, CT: Greenwood Press, 1983), 144.

7. Linda Kenney Miller, *Beacon on the Hill* (Marrietta, GA: Harper House Publishers, 2008), 158.

8. Thomas Ward, Jr., *Black Physicians in the Jim Crow South* (Fayetteville: University of Arkansas Press, 2003), 83.

"Clinic Note," *Journal of the National Medical Association* (January–March 1915), 58–59.

9. Beardsley, 150–151. Paul Cornelly, "Trends in Public Health Activities Among Negroes in 96 Southern Counties During the Period 1930–1939," *American Journal of Public Health* 32 (1942): 1123.

10. Chafe et al., 108.

11. P. Preston Reynolds, "Dr. Louis T. Wright and the NAACP: Pioneers in Hospital Racial Integration," *American Journal of Public Health* 90, no. 6 (June 2000): 996.

12. Lawrence O. Graham, *Our Kind of People* (New York: HarperCollins, 2000), 359.

13. Interview with Martie Elizabeth Branche Bauduit by Kelly Hughes, recorded on November 16, 2001, Maria Rogers Oral History Program, Carnegie Library.

14. Graham, 360.

Chapter 6

1. Vanessa N. Gamble, *Making a Place for Ourselves: The Black Hospital Movement, 1920–1945* (New York: Oxford University Press, 1995), 100; Clifton O. Dummett and Eugene Dibble, "Historical Notes on the Tuskegee Veterans Hospital," *Journal of the National Medical Association* 54, no. 2 (March 1952): 135.

2. Letter from John H. Ward to Louis T. Wright, July 28, 1924, Louis T. Wright Collection, Francis A. Countway Library of Medicine, Harvard Medical Library, Boston.

3. Pete Daniel, "Black Power in the 1920s: The Case of Tuskegee Veterans Hospital," *Journal of Southern History* 38 (1970): 368–388.

4. Dedication exercises of the Tuskegee Veterans Hospital Patient Rehabilitation and Recreation Program, June 25, 1927, TUA 329.004, folder 14, John A. Kenney Papers, Archives, Tuskegee University, Tuskegee, AL.

5. William T. B. Williams, "The World War & the Negro," *Southern Workman* 47 (1918): 519.

6. G. S. Moore, "An Introduction to a Study of Neuropsychiatric Problems among Negroes," *Veterans Bureau Medical Bulletin*, 1926 and 1927.

7. Letter from John Kenney to Booker T. Washington, in Booker T. Washington, *Booker T. Washington Papers*, 1914–1915, vol. 13 (Urbana: University of Illinois Press, 1984), 239–240.

8. Melvin J. Chisum, *The Faithful Narrative of an Investigation of the Tuskegee Veterans Hospital* (Chicago: National Negro Press Association, 1926), 1; TUA 329.004, folder 8, John A. Kenney Papers, Archives, Tuskegee University, Tuskegee, AL.

9. Herbert M. Morais, "The History of the Negro in Medicine," *The Association for the Study of Negro Life and History* (New York: Publications, Inc., 1967), 132.

10. Albion L. Holsey, "The Negro Veterans Hospital," *Southern Workman* 55 (1926): 313–314.

11. "Tuskegee, Alabama: The U.S. Veterans' Hospital," *Journal of the National Medical Association* 21 (1929): 65–67.

12. Annual Report of the State Board of Health of Alabama, 1930, 10–11.

13. Thomas Parran, *Shadow on the Land* (New York: Reynal & Hitchcock, 1937), 31–32.

14. Gamble, *Making a Place for Ourselves*, 54–55.

15. "Present Status of the Negro Physician and the Negro Patient," *Journal of the National Medical Association* XXVII (May 1935): 79.

16. Gamble, *Making a Place for Ourselves*, 103.

17. Williams, "The World War & the Negro."

18. Eugene Dibble, "Care and Treatment of Negro Veterans at Tuskegee," *Journal of the National Medical Association* (September 1943): 238.

19. George C. Branche, "Therapeutic

Chapter Notes—6

Quartan Malaria in the Treatment of Neurosyphilis among Negroes," *Journal of Nervous and Mental Disease* 83, no. 2 (February 1936): 177–188; "Therapeutic Quartan Malaria in the Treatment of Neurosyphilis Among Negroes," *American Journal of Psychiatry* 96 (1940): 967–978.

20. Robert White, "The Tuskegee Study of Untreated Syphilis Revisited," *Elsevier: The Lancet Infectious Disease* 6, no. 2 (February 2006): 62–63.

21. Theodore Rosengarten, *All God's Dangers: The Life of Nate Shaw* (New York: Knopf, 1974), 545.

22. Darlene Clark Hine, William C. Hine and Stanley Harrold, *The African-American Odyssey*, 4th ed. (Upper Saddle River, NJ: Prentice Hall, 2008), 482–483.

23. James H. Jones, *Bad Blood: The Tuskegee Syphilis Experiment* (New York: Free Press, 1993), 50–51.

24. Holmes, No. 625, S. 430. To amend Section 1106, code of Ala. 1923, relative to venereal disease control, Legislature of Alabama, passed at the Session of January 11, 1927.

25. Hine et al., *The African-American Odyssey*, 502–503.

26. Raymond A. Vonderlehr, "Introduction to the Tuskegee Study" (October 1964): 2. From the MS C264 documents on the origin and development of the Tuskegee Syphilis Study, 1921–1973, Box 1, Folder 35, C.D.C File M22–7, History of Medicine Division, National Library of Medicine, National Institutes of Health, Washington, D.C.

27. W. Montague Cobb, "The Tuskegee Syphilis Study," Briefs, *Journal of the National Medical Association* 65, no. 4 (July 1973): 346.

28. Paul A. Lombardo and Gregory M. Dorr, "Eugenics, Medical Education and the Public Health Service: Another Perspective on the Tuskegee Syphilis Experiment," *Bulletin of the History of Medicine* 80, no. 2 (Summer 2006): 291–316.

29. *Ibid.*, 313.

30. Thomas Parran, *Shadow on the Land: Syphilis* (New York: Reynal and Hitchcock, 1937), 175.

31. Meeting of Tuskegee researchers, April 5, 1965, MS C64 Documents, Box 1, Folder 36, C.D.C. File M22–7, History of Medicine Division, National Library of Medicine, Washington, D.C.

32. David Barton-Smith, *Health Care Divided: Race and Healing a Nation* (Ann Arbor: University of Michigan Press, 1990), 25–28.

33. *Final Report of The Tuskegee Syphilis Study Ad Hoc Advisory Panel*, U.S. Dept. of Health, Education & Welfare, Public Health Service, 1973, MS C264 Documents, Library of Medicine.

34. Letter from Austin V. Deibert to Raymond A. Vonderlehr, November 28, 1938.

35. Letter from Vonderlehr to Deibert, December 5, 1938.

36. R. G. James, *The Mobil Clinic and Syphilis in Macon County, Alabama*, 2–3, Box 2, Folder 44, C.D.C. File M25–21.

37. Barton-Smith, 83.

38. Jones, *Bad Blood*, 83; Susan E. Bell, "Events in the Tuskegee Syphilis Study, 1932–72: A Timeline," in Susan Reverby, *Examining Tuskegee* (Chapel Hill: University of North Carolina Press, 2009), 34.

39. Letter from Thomas Parran to Eugene Dibble, February 9, 1937, Box 1, Folder 42, C.D.C. File M25–30, Library of Medicine.

40. Letter from Dibble to Parran, February 12, 1938.

41. Stanley H. Schuman, Sidney Olansky, Eunice Rivers, C. A. Smith and Dorothy S. Rambo, "Untreated Syphilis in the Male Negro: Background and Current Status of Patients in the Tuskegee Study," *Journal of Chronic Diseases* 2, no. 6 (November 1955): 554–558.

42. Interview with James T. Braye, Tuskeege, Alabama, August 2008.

43. Stanley Olansky, *Outline for Tuskegee Study*, November 6, 1951, Box 2, Folder 47, C.D.C. File M25–13, Library of Medicine.

44. P. J. Pesare, *Report on Tuskegee Untreated Syphilis Study*, 1948, Box 2, Folder 46, C.D.C. File M25–12.
45. James, *The Mobil Clinic and Syphilis in Macon County, Alabama.*
46. Letter from Murray Smith to Raymond A. Vonderlehr, November 27, 1941, Box 1, Folder 28, C.D.C. File M25–3.
47. Letter from Seward Hilmer to Broadus Butler, October 29, 1972, Box 2, Folder 76, C.D.C. File M23–12.
48. Jones, *Bad Blood*, 208.
49. Letter from Vonderlehr to Smith, April 30, 1942, Box 1, Folder 30, C.D.C. File M22–3, Library of Medicine.
50. Letter from Smith to Vonderlehr, August 6, 1942.
51. Bill Jenkins, "The Tuskegee Study: A Study in Racism, Classism, and Medical Ethics," *AACOP Voice* 2, no. 3 (October 2004–February 2005): 1.
52. Final Report on the Tuskegee Syphilis Study Ad Hoc Advisory Panel.
53. Robert J. Norrell, *Reaping the Whirlwind: The Civil Rights Movement in Tuskegee* (New York: Alfred A. Knopf, 1985), 25.
54. *Ibid.*, 61–62.
55. James, *The Mobile Clinic and Syphilis in Macon County, Alabama*, 4.
56. Thomas Ward, *Black Physicians in the Jim Crow South* (Fayetteville: University of Arkansas Press, 2003), 39.
57. Eugene Dibble, "Care and Treatment of Negro Veterans at Tuskegee," *Journal of the National Medical Association* (September 1943): 235–236.
58. *Ibid.*, 236.
59. *The American Psychiatric Association Newsletter*, September 15, 1949, APA.
60. Dummitt and Dibble, "Historical Notes on the Tuskegee Veterans Hospital," 138.
61. Prince P. Barker, "Psychiatry at the Tuskegee VA Hospital in Retrospect," *Journal of The National Medical Association* 54, no. 2 (March 1962): 152.
62. Paul Cornely, "Trends in Public Health Activities Among Negroes in 96 Southern Counties During the Period, 1930–1939," *Journal of the American Public Health Association* 32 (1942): 1123.
63. William E. Alt and Betty L. Alt, *Black Soldiers, White Wars* (Westport, CT: Praeger, 2002), 91.
64. Gerald Astor, *The Right to Fight: A History of African Americans in the Military* (Novato, CA: Presido Press, 1998), 158–159.
65. Alt and Alt, 22.
66. Hine et al., *The African-American Odyssey*, 544.
67. Ronald H. Spector, *At War at Sea: Sailors and Naval Combat in the Twentieth Century* (New York: Viking, 2001), 265.
68. *Ibid.*, 170–171.
69. Howard W. Kenney and Julian W. Giles, "Tuskegee Veterans Administration Hospital—Present and Future," *Journal of the National Medical Association* 54 (March 1962): 136–137.
70. Philip McGuire, *Taps for a Jim Crow Army: Letters from Black Soldiers in World War II* (Santa Barbara: ABC-CLIO, 1983), 167–192.
71. Norrell, *Reaping the Whirlwind*, 46–48.
72. Lt. Col. (Ret.) Charles M. Bussey, *Firefight at Yechon: Courage and Racism in the Korean War* (Washington, D.C.: Brassey, 1991), 15.
73. Hine et al., 549.
74. Maj. Paul Goodman, *A Fragment of Victory: In Italy During World War II, 1944–45* (Carlisle, PA: Army War College, 1952), 5–7, 13.
75. Gamble, *Making a Place for Ourselves*, 185.
76. William T. Bowers, William M. Hammond, George L. MacGarrible, *Black Soldier—White Army* (Washington, D.C.: Center of Military History, United States Army, 1996), 37–38.
77. Norrell, *Reaping the Whirlwind*, 62–63.
78. *Ibid.*, 60–61.
79. Barker, "Psychiatry at the Tuskegee VA Hospital in Retrospect," 152.
80. Martin Binkin, *Blacks and the Military* (Washington, D. C.: Brookings Institution, 1986), 29.

Chapter 7

1. Clifton Dummett and Eugene H. Dibble, "Historical Notes on the Tuskegee Veterans Hospital," *Journal of the National Medical Association* 54, no. 2 (March 1962):133–138.

2. Herbert M. Morais, *The History of the Negro in Medicine* (New York: Publishers Company, 1967), pp. 178–179.

3. *Ibid.*, 184–185; "The Federal Government's Use of Title VI and Medicare to Racially Integrate Hospitals in the United States, 1963–1967," *American Journal of Public Health* 87 (November 1997): 1850–1858.

4. VA Hospital at Tuskegee Alabama Observes its 50th Year of Service, Congressional Record, March 1, 1973. From the MS C 264 Documents on the origin and development of the Tuskegee Syphilis Study, 1921–1973, Box 2, Folder 78, M60–9, History of Medicine Division, National Library of Medicine, National Institutes of Health, Washington, D.C.

5. Prince P. Barker, "Psychiatry at the Tuskegee VA Hospital in Retrospect," *Journal of the National Medical Association* 54, no. 2 (March 1962).

6. Vanessa Jackson, *Separate and Unequal: The Legacy of Racially Segregated Psychiatric Hospitals, a Culture Competence Training Tool*. Monograph accessed online, October 11, 2013. Atlanta: Healing Circles, 27.

7. Correspondence with Boston University Medical School Alumni Library, 2014.

8. Mary Kaplan, *Solomon Carter Fuller: Where My Caravan Has Rested* (Lanham, MD: University Press of America, 2005), 74.

9. *Ibid.*, 80.

10. *Ibid.*

11. Letter from Eugene Dibble to Solomon C. Fuller, from Solomon Carter Fuller's personal files.

12. James Jones, *Bad Blood: The Tuskegee Syphilis Experiment* (New York: Free Press, 1993), 217; Bill Jenkins, "The Tuskegee Study: A Study in Racism, Classism, and Medical Ethics," *AACOP Voice* 2, no. 3 (October 2004–February 2005): 1.

13. Vanessa N. Gamble, *Making a Place for Ourselves: The Black Hospital Movement, 1920–1945* (New York: Oxford University Press, 1995), 102.

Bibliography

Books

Alt, William E., and Betty L. Alt. *Black Soldiers, White Wars*. Westport, CT: Praeger, 2002.
Astor, Gerald. *The Right to Fight: A History of African Americans in the Military*. Novato, CA: Presido Press, 1998.
Bell, Leland V. *Treating the Mentally Ill*. Westport, CT: Praeger, 1980.
Binkin, Martin. *Blacks and the Military*. Washington, D.C.: Brookings Institution, 1986.
Bowers, William T., et al., *Black Soldier—White Army*. Washington, D.C.: Center of Military History, United States Army, 1996.
Briggs, Lloyd Vernon, ed. *A History of the Psychopathic Hospital*, Boston: Wright & Potter Printing Company, 1922.
Bussey, Lt. Col. (Ret.) Charles M. *Firefight at Yechon: Courage and Racism in the Korean War*. Washington, D.C.: Brassey, 2002.
Chafe, William, Raymond Gavins, and Robert Korstad, eds. *Remembering Jim Crow*. New York: The New Press, 2001.
Charles, Vert Willie, Bernard Kramer, and Bertram Brown, eds. *Racism and Mental Health*. Pittsburgh: University of Pittsburgh Press, 1973.
Cornish, Dudley T. *The Sable Arm: Negro Troops in the Union Army, 1861–1865*. New York: Norton, 1966.
Deutsch, Albert. *The Mentally Ill in America*. New York: Doubleday, 1938.
Dietrich, C., and C. Retzes, eds. *Negroes and Medicine*. Cambridge: The Commonwealth Fund, Harvard University Press, 1958.
Douglass, Frederick. *Life and Times of Frederick Douglas*. Reprinted from the revised edition of 1872. New York: Collier Books, 1962.
Eicher, David J. *The Longest Night: A Military History of the Civil War*. New York: Simon & Schuster, 2001.
Fraser, Walter J., and Winfred B. Moore, eds. *The Southern Enigma: Essays on Race, Class and Folk Culture*. Westport, CT: Greenwood Press, 1983.
Gamble, Vanessa N. *Making a Place for Ourselves: The Black Hospital Movement, 1920–1945*. New York: Oxford University Press, 1995.
Goodman, Maj. Paul. *A Fragment of Victory: In Italy During World War II, 1944–45*. Carlisle, PA: Army War College, 1952.

Bibliography

Graham, Lawrence O. *Our Kind of People*. New York: HarperCollins, 2000.

Hine, Darlene Clark, William C. Hine, and Stanley Harrold. *The African-American Odyssey*, 4th ed. Upper Saddle River, NJ: Prentice Hall, 2008.

Hughes, William H., and Frederick D. Patterson, eds. *Robert Russa Moton of Hampton and Tuskegee*. Chapel Hill: University of North Carolina Press, 1956.

Hurd, Henry M., et al. *The Institutional Care of the Insane in the United States and Canada, Vol. 1*. Baltimore: Johns Hopkins University Press, 1916.

Jay, David, and Elaine Crane. *The Black Soldier from the Revolution to Vietnam*. New York: William Morrow, 1971.

Jones, James. *Bad Blood: The Tuskegee Syphilis Experiment*. New York: Free Press, 1993.

Kaplan, H. Roy. *The Myth of Post-Racial America*. Lanham, MD: Rowman & Littlefield, 2011.

Kaplan, Mary. *Solomon Carter Fuller: Where My Caravan Has Rested*. Lanham, MD: University Press of America, 2005.

Kaplan, Sidney, and Emma Nogrady. *The Black Presence in the Era of the American Revolution*. Amherst: University of Massachusetts Press, 1989.

Litwack, Leon F. *Trouble in Mind: Black Southerners in the Age of Jim Crow*. New York: Alfred A. Knopf, 1998.

Marable, Manning, and Leith Mullins, eds. *Let Nobody Turn Us Around: Voices of Resistance, Reform, and Renewal: An African American Anthology*. Lanham, MD: Roman & Littlefield, 2000.

McCandless, Peter. *Moonlight, Magnolias and Madness: Insanity in South Carolina from the Colonial Period to the Progressive Era*. Chapel Hill: University of North Carolina Press, 1996.

McGuire, Philip. *Taps for a Jim Crow Army: Letters from Black Soldiers in World War II*. Santa Barbara, CA: ABC-CLIO, 1983.

Miller, Linda Kenney. *Beacon on the Hill*. Marrietta, GA: Harper House Publishers, 2008.

Morais, Herbert M. *The History of the Negro in Medicine*. New York: Publishers, 1967.

Nalty, Bernard C. *Strength for the Fights: A History of Black Americans in the Military*. New York: Free Press, 1986.

Nercessian, Nora. *Against All Odds: The Legacy of Students of African Descent at Harvard Medical School Before Affirmative Action, 1850–1968*. Boston: Puritan Press, 2004.

Norrell, Robert. *Reaping the Whirlwind: The Civil Rights Movement in Tuskegee*. New York: Alfred A. Knopf, 1985.

Parran, Thomas. *Shadow on the Land: Syphilis*. New York: Raynal & Hitchcock, 1937.

Reverby, Susan. *Examining Tuskegee*. Chapel Hill: University of North Carolina Press, 2000.

Roberts, James. *The Narrative of James Roberts, a Soldier Under General Washington in the Revolutionary War, and Under General Jackson at the Battle of New Orleans in the War of 1812: A Battle which Cost me a Limb, Some Blood and Almost My Life*, VII. Chicago: Printed for the author, 1858.

Bibliography

Rosengarten, Theodore. *All God's Dangers: The Life of Nate Shaw*. New York: Alfred A. Knopf, 1974.
Savitt, Todd. *Medicine and Slavery*. Urbana: University of Illinois Press, 1981.
Sharpley, Robert, ed. *Psychoanlysis, Psychotherapy, and the New England Medical Scene, 1844–1914*, New York: Science History Publishers, 1978.
Smith, David Barton. *Health Care Divided: Race and Healing a Nation*. Ann Arbor: University of Michigan Press, 1999.
Spector, Ronald H. *At War at Sea: Sailors and Naval Combat in the Twentieth Century*. New York: Viking, 2001.
Spurlock, Jeanne. *Black Psychiatrists and American Psychiatry*. Washington, D.C.: American Psychiatric Association, 1999.
Strecker, Edward A. "Military Psychiatry: World War I:, 1917–1918." *One Hundred Years of American Psychiatry*. New York: American Psychiatric Association and Columbia University Press, 1944.
Ward, Thomas. *Black Physicians in the Jim Crow South*. Fayetteville: University of Arkansas Press, 2003.
Washington, Booker T. *Booker T. Washington, 1914–1915*, vol. 13. Urbana: University of Illinois Press, 1984.
Wolters, Raymond. *The New Negro on Campus: Black College Rebellion of the 1920s*. Princeton: Princeton University Press, 1976.

Articles

Alexander, Caroline. "The Shock of War." *Smithsonian Magazine* 41, no. 5 (September 2010): 58–66.
"Alexander Thomas Augusta." *Journal of the National Medical Association* 44, no. 4 (July 1953): 328.
American Psychiatric Newsletter. September 15, 1949. American Psychiatric Association.
Amron, Andrew D. "Reinforcing Manliness: Black State Militias, The Spanish-American War, and the Image of the African American Soldier, 1891–1900." *The Journal of African American History* 97, no. 4 (Fall 2012).
Barker, Prince P. "Psychiatry at the Tuskegee VA Hospital in Retrospect." *Journal of the National Medical Association* 54, no. 2 (March 1962).
Bergman, Peter M. "The Negro who Rode with Fremont in 1847." *Negro History Bulletin* 28, no. 2.
Branche, George C. "Therapeutic Quartan Malaria in the Treatment of Neurosyphilis Among Negroes." *American Journal of Psychiatry* 96 (1940): 967–978.
_____. "Therapeutic Quartan Malaria in the Treatment of Neurosyphilis Among Negroes." *Journal of Nervous and Mental Disease* 83, no. 2 (February 1936): 177–188.
Brown, Scott. "White Backlash and the Aftermath of Fagen's Rebellion: The Fates of Three African American Soldiers in the Philippines, 1901–1902." *Contributions in Black Studies* 13, no. 5 (1995).
Buchanan, S. M. "Insanity in the Colored Race" *New York Medical Journal* 44 (1886): 69.

Bibliography

Cannon, George F. "The Negro Medical Profession and the United States Army." *Journal of the National Medical Association* 11, no. 1 (January–March 1919): 21–28.

Carter, James H. "Alcoholism in Black Vietnam Veterans: Symptoms of Post-Traumatic Stress Disorder." *Journal of the National Medical Association* 74, no. 7 (1983): 655.

"Clinic Note." *Journal of the National Medical Association* (January–March 1915): 58–59.

Cobb, W. Montague. "The Tuskegee Syphilis Study." *Journal of the National Medical Association* 65, no. 4 (July 1973): 346.

Cornelly, Paul. "Trends in Public Health Activities Among Negroes in 96 Southern Counties During the Period 1930–1939." *American Journal of Public Health* 32 (1942): 1123.

Daniel, Pete. "Black Power in the 1920s: the Case of the Tuskegee Veterans Hospital." *Journal of Southern History* 36, no. 3 (August 1970): 368–388.

Dibble, Eugene. "Care and Treatment of Negro Veterans at Tuskegee." *Journal of the National Medical Association* (September 1943): 238.

DuBois, W. E. B. "No Compromise." *The Crisis* 72 (November 1923).

———. "Opinion: The Tuskegee Hospital." *The Crisis* 26 (July 1923): 106–107.

———. "Reconstruction and its Benefits." *American Historical Review* 15 (1910).

Dummett, Clifton, and Eugene H. Dibble. "Historical Notes on the Tuskegee Veterans Hospital." *Journal of the National Medical Association* LIV, no. 52 (March 1962): 135.

Flexner, Abraham, and Henry Pritchett. "Medical Education in the United States and Canada." *Carnegie Foundation for the Advancement of Teaching*, Bulletin 4 (1910): 180.

Freeman, Elsie, Wynell B. Schamel, and Jean West. "The Fight for Equal Rights: A Recruiting Poster for Black Soldiers in the Civil War." *Social Education* 56, no. 2 (February 1992).

"A French Directive." *The Crisis* 18 (May 1919).

Gatewood, William B. "Alabama's Negro Soldier Experience, 1898–1899." *Journal of Negro History* 57 (October 1972).

Green, E. M. "Manic-Depressive Psychoses in the Negro." *American Journal of Insanity* 73 (1917): 619–626.

Grimsley, Mark. "Confederate Rage, Yankee Wrath—No Quarter in the Civil War." *Civil War History*, 55, no 3 (2009): 414–415.

Grob, Gerald. "Class, Ethnicity and Race in American Mental Hospitals." *Journal of the History of Medicine* 28 (1973): 207–229.

Groves, Harry. "Separate but Equal—The Doctrine of Plessy v Ferguson." *Phylon* 12, no. 1.

Holsey, Albion L. "The Negro Veterans' Hospital." *The Southern Workmen* 52 (July 1926).

"Hospital for Ex-Servicemen to be at Tuskegee." *Journal of the National Medical Association* (1922).

Jenkins, Bill. "The Tuskegee Study: A Study in Racism, Classism, and Medical Ethics." *AACOP Voice*, 2, no. 3 (October 2004–February 2005): 1.

Bibliography

Kenney, Howard W., and Julian W. Giles. "Tuskegee Veterans Administration Hospital—Present and Future." *Journal of the National Medical Association* 54 (March 1962): 132–137.

Kenney, John. "A Shortage of Negro Doctors: With Special Reference to Residents and Interns." *Annual Bulletin, John A. Andrews Clinic.* Tuskegee Institute, 1940, 85.

Lombardo, Paul, and Gregory M. Dorr. "Eugenics, Medical Education and the Public Health Service: Another Perspective on the Tuskegee Syphilis Experiment." *Bulletin of the History of Medicine* 80, no. 2 (Summer 2006): 291–316.

Moore, G. S. "An Introduction to a Study of Neuropsychiatric Problems Among Negroes." *Veterans Bureau Medical Bulletin* 1926 and 1927.

Morais, Herbert M. "The Federal Government's Use of Title VI and Medicare to Racially Integrate Hospitals in the United States, 1963–1967." *American Journal of Public Health* 87 (November 1997): 1850–1858.

"Negro Doctors and Hospitals." *Opportunity* 3 (1925): 227.

O'Malley, Mary. "Psychoses in the Colored Race." *American Journal of Insanity* 73 (1917): 326–327.

"Present Status of the Negro Physician and the Negro Patient." *Journal of the National Medical Association* XXVII (May 1935): 79.

Reynolds, P. Preston. "Dr. Louis T. Wright and the NAACP: Pioneers in Hospital Racial Integration." *American Journal of Public Health* 90, no. 6 (June 2000): 996.

Schuman, Stanley H., et al. "Untreated Syphilis in the Male Negro: Background and Current Status of Patients in the Tuskegee Study." *Journal of Chronic Diseases* 2, no. 6 (November 1956): 554–556.

Summers, Martin. "Suitable Care of the African When Afflicted with Insanity: Race, Madness, and Social Order in Comparative Perspective." *Bulletin of the History of Medicine* 84, no. 1 (Spring 2010): 66–67.

"Tuskegee, Alabama: The U. S. Veterans' Hospital." *Journal of the National Medical Association* 21 (1929): 65–67.

"The Tuskegee Hospital Muddle." *The Crisis* 28 (September 1923).

The Tuskegee Student. March 1–15, 1923.

White, Robert. "The Tuskegee Study of Untreated Syphilis Revisited." *Elsevier: The Lancet Infectious Disease* 6, no. 2 (February 2006): 62–63.

Williams, William T. B. "The World War & the Negro." *Southern Workman* 47 (1918): 519.

Wright, Louis T. "The New Doctor and the War." *Journal of the National Medical Association* 11, no. 4 (1951): 96.

Younge, Samuel L. *Journal of the National Medical Association* 56, no. 6 (1965): 565–566.

Government Documents, Reports and Collections

Annual Report of the State Board of Health of Alabama, 1930.

Consultants on Hospitalization, Record Group 121, Records of the Public Building Service, National Archives, Washington, D.C.

Bibliography

Documents on the origin and development of the Tuskegee Syphilis Study, 1921–1973, Collection Number: MS C 264. Manuscripts Collection, History of Medicine Division, National Library of Medicine, United States, Department of Health, Education, and Welfare, Bethesda, MD.

McClure, Barbara. "Medical Care Programs of the Veterans Administration." *Congressional Research Service Report No. 83–99*, Library of Congress, Washington, D.C., May 1983.

Militia Act of 1792, United States at Large, Vol. 1, United States Congress, Public Acts of the Second Congress, First Session, Chapter 33.

Robert Moton Papers, Boxes 71, 95, File: Government Hospital 700, National Archives, Washington, D.C.

The National Association for the Advancement of Colored People (NAACP) Papers, Group I, Series C410, Container 410, Library of Congress, Washington, D.C.

Smith, Steven D. and Zeidler, James A. (Eds.) "A Historic Context for the African American Military Experience." United States Army Construction Engineering Research Laboratories, July 1998.

Union and Confederate Armies Official Records, Series IV, Vol. III. Washington, D.C.: Government Printing Office, 1900.

Scholarly Papers and Publications

Cetina, Judith G. *A History of Veterans Homes in the United States, 1811–1930*. Ph.D. dissertation, Case Western Reserve University, 1977.

Fuller, Solomon Carter. "Anatomical Findings of General Paresis and Multiple Sclerosis in the Same Case." S. C. Fuller Personal File (date unknown).

Ryff, Alan W. "The Tuskegee Hospital Controversy, 1921–1924." M.A. Thesis, University of Delaware, 1970.

Archives

Francis A. Countway Library of Medicine, Harvard Medical Library, Boston. Louis T. Wright Collection.

Tuskegee Archives, Tuskegee University, Tuskegee, Alabama. John A. Kenney Papers, Box 329.04, Folders 8, 14. Robert Moton Papers, Box 90, File: 669, Box 95, File: Government Hospital 700, Box 125, File: 941

Newspapers

Atlanta Independent, Editorial, May 24, 1923
Baltimore Afro-American, August 31, 1923
Mobile Register, July 5, 1923
Montgomery Advertiser, July 4, 1923
New York Age, July 21, 1923
New York Herald, June 16, 1918
Norfolk Pilot, July 21, 1923
Savannah Tribune, July 4, 1923

Bibliography

Internet

"The Brownsville Affair." Dictionary of American History, www.encylopedia.com.
Christian, Gama L. "Brownsville Raid of 1906." The Handbook of Texas Online, Texas State Historical Association, www.tshaonline.org.
"History of the National Home for Disabled Volunteer Soldiers." National Park Service, United States Department of the Interior, www.nps.gov.
Interview with Martie Elizabeth Branche Bauduit by Kelly Hughes. Recorded on November 16, 2001, Maria Rogers Oral History Program, Carnegie Library, www.oralhistoryboulderlibrary.org/interview/oh1130.
Lord Dunmore's Proclamation. Digital History, http://digitalhistory.uh.edu/learninghistory/revolution/dunmore.com.
"VA History in Brief." Department of Veterans Affairs, www.va.gov.cpa/publications/archives/docs/history.

Index

Aborigines (Liberia) 11–12
Academie Colarossi 45
Acley, Miss 44–45
Adams, George 21–22, 25
Adler, Alfred 52, 60
Allentown State Hospital (Pennsylvania) 53, 73
Alzheimer, Alois 35, 36–38, 50, 56–58
American Art Student's Club for Women (Paris) 44–45
American Colonization Society (ACS) 4–5, 7, 12
American Girl's Club *see* American Art Student's Club for Women (Paris)
American Medical Association 68, 75
American Medico-Psychological Association 22, 26–27
American Methodist Episcopal Church 15, 17
American Psychiatric Association 65, 80
American Society for Colonizing Free People of Color in the United States *see* American Colonization Society (ACS)
Americo-Liberians 11–12
Angelou, Maya vii
L'Art Nouveau (Parisian art salon) 46
Ashmun, Jehudi 7–8
Atlantic City 27, 43, 47
Auguste, D. 37
Ayer, James 76

Baker, Dr. 25
Baltimore 8
Barclay, Arthur 33, 70
Barclay, Sara 33
Belding 56
Belleview Hospital Medical College 28

Bent, Arthur 50
Betts 57
Biggs, Hermann 28
Bing, Samuel 46
Bioko, Equatorial Guinea *see* Fernando Po
Black Psychiatrists of America 80
Blocq 57
Board of Donations for Education (Liberia) 18–19
Bollinger, Otto 35
Boston Medical Center vii
Boston Psychopathic Hospital 18
Boston Stock Exchange 69
Boston Symphony 63
Boston University 27; Division of Psychiatry 80; Medical Center 79; School of Medicine 18, 21, 26, 29, 41, 53, 64, 65, 67–68, 80
Boundary Commission of Liberia 11
Boy Scouts of America 69
Bragg, Evan 29
Bragg, Mary (May) *see* Weston, Mary (May) Bragg
Branche, George 65
Brooklyn, New York 48
Brown, Auntie 50
Brown, Margaret 47
Brown, Nancy 5
Brush, Edward 52
Burleigh, Harry 63

Calderon, Pablo 81
Caldwell (Liberia) 12
Calloway, Thomas 45
Campbell, Macfie 65
Carles, Antoine 45
Carnegie Institute 28

Index

Cartier, Alexander 47
cassada 9
Catskill Mountains, New York 17
Charitable Mechanics Society (Boston) 9
Clark Celebration 51
Clark University (Worcester, Massachusetts) 50–52
Clarke 57
Clay, Henry 4
Clinical Society Commission of Massachusetts 26
Colby, Edward P. 21–22
Colby College 68, 74
Coles, Dr. 31
College Preparatory School (Monrovia) 13
Collin, Raphael 45
Colored Episcopal Church, Atlantic City 47
Congoes 11
Councilman, W.T. 39, 55–56
cran-cran 9
Crane, Stephen 46
The Crisis 59, 65
Cushing, Harvey 53
Cushing Hospital (Framingham) 77

Davis, Harvey 65
Deaver, Rev. Mr. 47
Democratic Party 75
Dr. Solomon Carter Fuller Mental Health Center vii-viii, 79–80
DuBois, W.E.B. 42, 58–59, 62
Dunford, Judith 1
Dunham, Edward K. 28, 36, 38

Earhart, Amelia 70
Ecole des Beaux Arts 45
Edinger, Ludwig 38
Ehrlich, Paul 38–40, 55
Eisenhower, Dwight 75
Elizabeth, New Jersey 69
Ellison, Ralph ix
Elmwood Opera House (Framingham) 49
Emancipation Proclamation 59
Episcopal Church, Atlantic City 47
Equal Suffrage Movement 70
Ethiopia Awakening 46

Fair Employment Practices Commission 75

Fay, Harold 63
Ferenczi, Sandor 51
Fernando Po 71
Firestone Company 11, 71
Fischer 57
Fisk Jubilee Singers 44
Framingham, Massachusetts 49–50, 54, 72, 76, 77, 81
Framingham Dramatic Club 63
Framingham South High School *see* Fuller Middle School
Framingham Union Hospital 76
Framingham's Women's Club 77
Frankfort, Germany 38–40
Freud, Sigmund 50, 51, 60
Fuller, Anna Ursula James 10–11, 33, 71
Fuller, Harriet 83–84
Fuller, Henry 3, 10
Fuller, John Lewis (grandfather of SCF) xiv, 1–5, 7–10, 84
Fuller, John Lewis (grandson of SCF) xv, 73–74
Fuller, John Lewis, Jr. 3
Fuller, Margaret 3
Fuller, Meta Vaux Warrick *see* Warrick, Meta Vaux
Fuller, Nancy (daughter of John Lewis Fuller) *see* Jarratt, Nancy Fuller
Fuller, Nancy (wife of John Lewis Fuller) 2–3, 5
Fuller, Perry James 62, 68–70
Fuller, Rebecca 3, 8
Fuller, Sarah 3, 5
Fuller, Solomon (father of SCF) 3, 5, 8, 10–14
Fuller, Solomon Carter: attitudes toward wife's art career 62, 76; birth 10; blindness and old age 73–75; death and funeral services 76; early relationship with and marriage to Meta Vaux Warrick 42, 46–48; education at Boston University 18–21; education at Livingstone College, North Carolina 15–17; education in Liberia 12–14; friends in later years 72–73; home and visitors in Framingham 49–50, 62–63; internship at Westboro Insane Hospital 22–24; military and veteran-related activities 60–62, 64–65, 75; pathologist at Westboro 24–31, 41–42, 55–56; post-graduate education in Munich

Index

xiii-xv, 30–38; psychiatric practice 60; relationship to family in Liberia 70–71; relationship to sons 63, 68–69; religious beliefs 71–72; research and publication 56–58, 59; retirement from Boston University 67–68; visit to Frankfort 38–40; visits by Liberians 71

Fuller, Solomon Carter, Jr. x, xiv-xv, 53–55 passim, 60–63 passim, 68–69, 72–76 passim, 79, 81 passim

Fuller, Thomas (uncle of SCF) 3, 5, 10

Fuller, Thomas George (brother of SCF) 11, 70–71

Fuller, William Thomas (Tom) 58, 68–69, 73, 76

Fuller Middle School 81

Gibraltar 33–34
Gibson 13
Goldman, Emma 51
Gorman Theatre (Framingham) 49
Grace Church (Framingham) 70
Graham, Lawrence Otis 49
Greenwich Village 69

Haines, Thomas 13
Hall, G. Stanley 50–51
Harding Administration 64
Harlem 69
Harnack, Adolf von 34
Harriet Tubman Square Park 59
Harvard Medical School 39, 55–56, 66, 72, 80
Hayden Scholarship 18
Hayes, Roland 63
Hemings, Fred 47
Hemings, Sally 10, 47
Henderson, Alfred R. ix-x
Herter, Christian A. 28
Hilton, Frances 13
Hines, General 65
Hinton, William 72
Hodes, J. Allison 26
Hodge, Professor 51
Holt, L. Emmett 30
Hoover, Velma 59
Hospital for Sick and Injured Colored War Veterans *see* Tuskegee Veterans Hospital
Howard University 76
Hurd, Henry Mills 52

Imperial Institute for Chemical Research, Frankfort 38
Isaacs, Harold R. 67

J. Liberty Tadd (Philadelphia art school) 44
James, Anna Ursula *see* Fuller, Anna Ursula James
James, Benjamin Van Rensalaer 10–11
James, Commodore 10
James, William 53
Jamestown Tercentennial Exposition 46–47
Jansen 58
Jarratt, Alexander 2–3
Jarratt, Nancy Fuller 2–3
Jarratt family 17, 48
jiggers 9
Johann Wolfgang Goethe University 37
Johns Hopkins Medical School 24, 28, 30, 52
Johnson, Elijah 7
Johnson, Simon 65
Jones, Emma *see* Warrick, Emma Jones.
Jones, Henry 43
Joslin Diabetes Center (Boston) 73
Jung, Carl 51, 52, 60

Keene, New Hampshire 72–73
Kennedy School of Government (Harvard University) 83
King, Charles D.B. 71
King, Charles H., Jr. 21
King, Drue 65
Klopp, Henry 28, 53
Knight, E.G. 47
Koch, Robert 28
Kraepelin, Emil xiii, 30, 35, 38, 41, 50, 52, 57
Ku Klux Klan 60

Lafora 58
Larner's Pond 70
Lewy, Frederick H. 37
Liberia 5, 7–14, 18–19, 33, 70–71; *see also* Monrovia, Liberia
Liberia College 13–14
Livingstone College (Salisbury, NC) 15–17, 75, 77
Long Branch, New Jersey 17
Long Island College Hospital 17–18

149

Index

Loudin, Frederick 44
Loudin, Harriet 44

Mahl, Professor 24
Mallory 56, 57–58
Man Eating His Heart 46, 54
Manhattan Beach Hotel 18
Marlboro Hospital (Framingham) 53, 73
Martha's Vineyard Sound 76, 77
Mary Turner 46
Maryland (Liberia) 10, 11
Massachusetts Clinical Society Commission 53
Massachusetts Department of Mental Health v
Massachusetts Legislature 79
Massachusetts Memorial Hospital 53, 64
Massachusetts State Board of Insanity 52
Massachusetts State Hospital for the Insane *see* Westborough State Hospital
Max Planck Institute of Psychiatry 35
Mechanics Charitable Society (Monrovia) 9
Mellis, Edward 22, 23–24, 30
Menninger, Karl 66
Menninger Clinic 66
Merriam, John 49
Merrill Lynch 69
Meyer, Adolf 50, 52, 53
Middlesex County Sanitarium 76
Mitchell, S. Weir 22–23
Monroe, James 7
Monrovia, Liberia 5, 7, 33, 70; *see also* Liberia
Mt. Moriah Cemetery, Philadelphia 43
Munich Psychiatric Hospital 35
Murray Hill Hotel, New York 17

National Association for the Advancement of Colored People (NAACP) 58–59, 64, 75, 77
National Medical Association 64, 80
New England Medical Gazette 29
"New Vistas in American Art" exhibition 76
New York City 28, 70
New York University School of Medicine 28
Newport, Rhode Island 64
Newport Yacht Club 10, 64
Niagara Movement 42

Nimmo (or Nimo), Rebecca 5, 13
Norfolk, Virginia 1–5
North Carolina 15–17

Overholser, Winfred 65–66

Page, Naida Willette 80
Paris Exposition of 1899 45
Paris Exposition of 1900 45
Peace Halting the Ruthlessness of War 62
Pennsylvania College of Art *see* Philadelphia School of Industrial Art
Pentagon 83
Peter Brent Brigham Hospital (Boston) 53
Petersburg, Virginia 1–2
Philadelphia 43–44, 54, 69
Philadelphia Academy of Fine Arts 44
Philadelphia Academy of Music 43
Philadelphia School of Industrial Art 44
Pierce, Pr. 10
Pinderhughes, Charles 74, 80
Plaut, Felix 35
Price, Joseph Charles 16
Price Memorial Building (Livingstone College) 75
The Procession of Arts and Crafts 44
Prudhomme, Charles 80
Psychiatric Hospital (Boston) 65

Randolph, A. Philip 75
"Red Summer" (1919) 60
Reid, Mrs. Whitelaw 45
Reiss, Edward 35
Roberts, Joseph Jenkins 7, 8
Robeson, Paul 63
Rockefeller Institute 28, 30
Rodin, Auguste 46
Rodriguez, Juan 81
Roosevelt, Franklin 65, 75
Roosevelt, Theodore 47

St. Andrew's Episcopal Church (Framingham) 77
St. Elizabeth's Psychiatric Hospital (Washington, DC) 65
Saint-Gaudens, Augustus 45
St. Stephen's Church (Framingham) 60
St. Thomas Church (Philadelphia) 47
Schmaus, Hans 35–36
Senckenberg Institute 38

Index

September 11, 2001 attack on Pentagon 83
Sharply, Robert H. 80
Sheepshead Bay 18
Sherbrook 7
Shredded Wheat Company 47
Sidney, Maine 29
Sierra Leone 7, 11
Sierra Leone Mountains 34
sleeping disease 9
"Solomon Carter Fuller Day" 80
Solomon Fuller Institute 80
Sousa, John Philip 18
South-West German Alienists 37
Southard, Elmer 18, 56
Southwest German Psychiatric Society 57
Spirit of Emancipation 59
Stanley, Robert C. 64
Star of Zion 17
State Reform School for Boys (Massachusetts) 21
Stewart, Margaret 10–11
Submarine Signal Company 63
Supreme Court 75
Sutherland, John P. 25, 65
Syphilis and Its Treatment 72

Talented Tenth 42
Tanner, Henry O. 44–45
Tildon, Toussaint T. 65
Townsend, the Rev. Mr. 47
Trent, William J. 77
Truman, Harry 75
Tuskegee, Alabama 64
Tuskegee Air Base 69
Tuskegee Institute 64
Tuskegee Veterans Hospital 64–65
Tyzzer, Ernest 39

United Community Services (Boston) 69
United States Armed Forces 64
United States Army, Secretary of 83
United States Veterans' Bureau 64–65
University of Munich xi, 30, 35

Vaux, Richard 43
Ventnor, New Jersey 43
Veterans Administration *see* United States Veterans' Bureau
Virchow, Rudolf 22
Voit, Karl von 35

von Harnack, Adolf *see* Harnack, Adolf von
von Voit, Karl *see* Voit, Karl von

Waller, Meta Louis Fuller 83–84
War Department 61–62
Warren, President (Carnegie Institute) 36
Ward, Dr. 74
Warrick, Blanche 44
Warrick, Emma Jones 43, 44
Warrick, Meta Vaux: ancestry, birth, and early childhood 43; art education in the United States 44; birth of son Perry 62; birth of son Solomon, Jr. 54; birth of son Tom 58; bust of SCF 79; community, religious, and political activities 63, 70, 72, 76–77, 81; death 77; early relationship with and marriage to Solomon Carter Fuller 42, 46–48; friendship with W.E.B. DuBois 45–46; home in Framingham 49–50, 54; loss of artwork to fire 54; postgraduate study in Paris 44–46; return to art activities 58–59, 62–63, 70, 72, 76–77
Warrick, William H. 43, 44
Washington, Booker T. 16, 42
Webster, Thomas 66
Weigert, Carl 38
Weiler, Karl 35
Welch, William Henry 28
West Virginia State College 74
Westboro Insane Hospital *see* Westborough State Hospital
Westborough (or *Westboro*) *State Hospital Papers* 29, 59
Westborough State Hospital (originally Westboro Insane Hospital) 21–31, 36, 52–53, 56, 59, 64, 73
Weston, Arthur 72–73
Weston, Mary (May) Bragg 29–30, 68, 72–73, 76
Weston, Ruth 72–73
Williams, Frankwood E. 61–62
Women's Peace Party 62, 70
Wood, Harry 17
Worcester State Hospital 50
World War I 60–62, 64, 75
World War II 75
The Wretched 54
Wright, Clarence W. 75
Wright, Louis T. 65

YMCA (Harlem) 69

151

www.ingramcontent.com/pod-product-compliance
Ingram Content Group UK Ltd.
Pitfield, Milton Keynes, MK11 3LW, UK
UKHW042017140426
5217IPUK00015B/1219

9 781476 662985